SpringerBriefs in Sociology

SpringerBriefs in Sociology are concise summaries of cutting-edge research and practical applications across the field of sociology. These compact monographs are refereed by and under the editorial supervision of scholars in Sociology or cognate fields. Volumes are 50 to 125 pages (approximately 20,000- 70,000 words), with a clear focus. The series covers a range of content from professional to academic such as snapshots of hot and/or emerging topics, in-depth case studies, and timely reports of state-of-the art analytical techniques. The scope of the series spans the entire field of Sociology, with a view to significantly advance research. The character of the series is international and multi-disciplinary and will include research areas such as: health, medical, intervention studies, cross-cultural studies, race/class/gender, children, youth, education, work and organizational issues, relationships, religion, ageing, violence, inequality, critical theory, culture, political sociology, social psychology, and so on. Volumes in the series may analyze past, present and/or future trends, as well as their determinants and consequences. Both solicited and unsolicited manuscripts are considered for publication in this series. SpringerBriefs in Sociology will be of interest to a wide range of individuals, including sociologists, psychologists, economists, philosophers, health researchers, as well as practitioners across the social sciences. Briefs will be published as part of Springer's eBook collection, with millions of users worldwide. In addition, Briefs will be available for individual print and electronic purchase. Briefs are characterized by fast, global electronic dissemination, standard publishing contracts, easy-to-use manuscript preparation and formatting guidelines, and expedited production schedules. We aim for publication 8-12 weeks after acceptance.

Uwe Engel
Editor

Robots in Care and Everyday Life

Future, Ethics, Social Acceptance

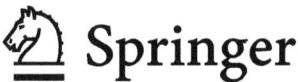 Springer

Editor
Uwe Engel
Department of Social Sciences
University of Bremen
Bremen, Germany

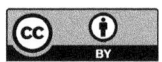

ISSN 2212-6368　　　　　　　ISSN 2212-6376　(electronic)
SpringerBriefs in Sociology
ISBN 978-3-031-11446-5　　　ISBN 978-3-031-11447-2　(eBook)
https://doi.org/10.1007/978-3-031-11447-2

© The Author(s) 2023. This book is an open access publication.
Open Access This book is licensed under the terms of the Creative Commons Attribution 4.0 International License (http://creativecommons.org/licenses/by/4.0/), which permits use, sharing, adaptation, distribution and reproduction in any medium or format, as long as you give appropriate credit to the original author(s) and the source, provide a link to the Creative Commons license and indicate if changes were made.
The images or other third party material in this book are included in the book's Creative Commons license, unless indicated otherwise in a credit line to the material. If material is not included in the book's Creative Commons license and your intended use is not permitted by statutory regulation or exceeds the permitted use, you will need to obtain permission directly from the copyright holder.
The use of general descriptive names, registered names, trademarks, service marks, etc. in this publication does not imply, even in the absence of a specific statement, that such names are exempt from the relevant protective laws and regulations and therefore free for general use.
The publisher, the authors, and the editors are safe to assume that the advice and information in this book are believed to be true and accurate at the date of publication. Neither the publisher nor the authors or the editors give a warranty, expressed or implied, with respect to the material contained herein or for any errors or omissions that may have been made. The publisher remains neutral with regard to jurisdictional claims in published maps and institutional affiliations.

This Springer imprint is published by the registered company Springer Nature Switzerland AG
The registered company address is: Gewerbestrasse 11, 6330 Cham, Switzerland

Preface

Artificial intelligence represents a key technology that is already changing the world today, with the expectation of changing the world in much more fundamental ways in the future. The widespread reluctance of sociology to deal with this challenge is more than astonishing. We still observe a lack of methodologically trustworthy data from social research. For example, the European Social Survey, the flagship of European social research, has not provided any such data to date; Eurobarometer studies do occasionally provide at least some smaller question modules. That is not much.

Thus, we wanted to contribute to closing this research gap by providing thematically more extensive and differentiated survey data, even if this were only possible in a local sample of the Free Hanseatic City of Bremen. But we also wanted to help close an additional research gap. The key questions were: In what way will AI change society, and how will the interaction with robots change people's everyday life? Although we cannot provide precise forecasts, we can show which developments experts do expect, from today's perspective. For this, we used the Delphi method, asking a larger selection of experts from different disciplines for their scientific assessments.

A sociological investigation at the intersection of AI and society certainly runs the risk of one-sided alarmism, nor would that be completely unpopular. However, to avoid any one-sidedness from the outset, we paid much attention to professional heterogeneity, in terms of the constituency of experts that we asked for their opinions and the project group itself. This latter group is affiliated with two major institutions at the Bremen science location, the Robotics Innovation Center, Deutsches Forschungszentrum für Künstliche Intelligenz GmbH (DFKI), and diverse chairs of the University of Bremen. As the context of each chapter details, these institutions involve the Robotics Chair and EASE, the Bremen Spatial Cognition Center, the Civil Law Chair, and the Social Science Methods Centre. The scientific backgrounds of the project members represent robotics, cognition science, jurisprudence, and social science.

The idea for the "Bremen AI Delphi" project was born in the context of the Digital Traces Workshop, which took place on November 8–10, 2018, at the University of Bremen. The Social Science Methods Centre organized the three-day workshop, and the German Research Foundation (DFG), the federal state of Bremen, and the Bremen International Graduate School of Social Sciences funded it. During the workshop, an interdisciplinary group of scholars shared recent advancements in computational social science and established new research collaborations. Questionnaire construction and fielding were realized in 2019. A first major report to the public took place on a project-related "theme day" at Radio Bremen on January 14, 2020, four weeks after the end of the field phase. With this volume, we present the project's major findings for scientific discussion.

The grand financial support of the State and University Library Bremen (SuUB) enables free access to this book. We are extremely grateful to SuUB for this support.

Bremen, Germany
January 27, 2022

Uwe Engel

Contents

1 **Trustworthiness and Well-Being: The Ethical, Legal, and Social Challenge of Robotic Assistance** 1
Michael Beetz, Uwe Engel, Nina Hoyer, Lorenz Kähler, Hagen Langer, Holger Schultheis, and Sirko Straube

2 **Artificial Intelligence and the Labor Market: Expected Development and Ethical Concerns in the German and European Context** 27
Uwe Engel and Lena Dahlhaus

3 **The Bremen AI Delphi Study** 49
Uwe Engel and Lena Dahlhaus

4 **The Challenge of Autonomy: What We Can Learn from Research on Robots Designed for Harsh Environments** 57
Sirko Straube, Nina Hoyer, Niels Will, and Frank Kirchner

5 **The Legal Challenge of Robotic Assistance** 81
Lorenz Kähler and Jörn Linderkamp

6 **Cognition-Enabled Robots Assist in Care and Everyday Life: Perspectives, Challenges, and Current Views and Insights** 103
Michael Beetz, Uwe Engel, and Hagen Langer

7 **Ethical Challenges of Assistive Robotics in the Elderly Care: Review and Reflection** 121
Mona Abdel-Keream

Contributors

Mona Abdel-Keream University of Bremen, Bremen, Germany

Michael Beetz University of Bremen, Bremen, Germany

Lena Dahlhaus University of Oldenburg, Oldenburg, Germany

Uwe Engel University of Bremen, Bremen, Germany

Nina Hoyer Robotics Research Group, University of Bremen, Bremen, Germany
Robotics Innovation Center, Deutsches Forschungszentrum für Künstliche Intelligenz GmbH (DFKI), Bremen, Germany

Lorenz Kähler University of Bremen, Bremen, Germany

Frank Kirchner Robotics Innovation Center, Deutsches Forschungszentrum für Künstliche Intelligenz GmbH (DFKI), Bremen, Germany
Robotics Research Group, University of Bremen, Bremen, Germany

Hagen Langer University of Bremen, Bremen, Germany

Jörn Linderkamp University of Bremen, Bremen, Germany

Holger Schultheis University of Bremen, Bremen, Germany

Sirko Straube Robotics Innovation Center, Deutsches Forschungszentrum für Künstliche Intelligenz GmbH (DFKI), Bremen, Germany

Niels Will Robotics Innovation Center, Deutsches Forschungszentrum für Künstliche Intelligenz GmbH (DFKI), Bremen, Germany

Chapter 1
Trustworthiness and Well-Being: The Ethical, Legal, and Social Challenge of Robotic Assistance

Michael Beetz, Uwe Engel, Nina Hoyer, Lorenz Kähler, Hagen Langer, Holger Schultheis, and Sirko Straube

Abstract If a technology lacks social acceptance, it cannot realize dissemination into society. The chapter thus illuminates the ethical, legal, and social implications of robotic assistance in care and daily life. It outlines a conceptual framework and identifies patterns of trust in human–robot interaction. The analysis relates trust in robotic assistance and its anticipated use to open-mindedness toward technical innovation and reports evidence that this self-image unfolds its psychological impact on accepting robotic assistance through the imagined well-being that scenarios of future human–robot interaction evoke in people today. All findings come from the population survey of the Bremen AI Delphi study.

Keywords Artificial intelligence · AI · Robots · Robotic assistance · Trust · Trustworthiness · Social acceptance · Ethics · Human–robot interaction · Well-being · Care · Everyday life

1.1 Introduction

That artificial intelligence and robots will change life is widely expected. International competition alone will ensure continuing investments in this key technology. No country will be able to maintain its economic competitiveness if it does not invest

M. Beetz · U. Engel (✉) · L. Kähler · H. Langer · H. Schultheis
University of Bremen, Bremen, Germany
e-mail: uengel@uni-bremen.de

N. Hoyer
University of Bremen, Bremen, Germany

Robotics Innovation Center, Deutsches Forschungszentrum für Künstliche Intelligenz GmbH (DFKI), Bremen, Germany

S. Straube
Robotics Innovation Center, Deutsches Forschungszentrum für Künstliche Intelligenz GmbH (DFKI), Bremen, Germany

© The Author(s) 2023
U. Engel (ed.), *Robots in Care and Everyday Life*, SpringerBriefs in Sociology,
https://doi.org/10.1007/978-3-031-11447-2_1

in research and the development of such a key technology. However, this premise complicates things if AI applications do not meet with the necessary acceptance in a country's society, including acceptance by social interest groups and, thus, acceptance in the population. Populations in democratically constituted, liberal societies using to a greater extent technologies that they do not want to use is a difficult scenario to imagine.

This raises the question of AI's social and ethical acceptance. How should the development of this technology advance to gain and secure this acceptance? The key lies in the perceived trustworthiness of the technology and, consequently, the reasons that lead people and interest groups to attest to this property of AI and its applications. For instance, as the Royal Society (2017) puts it, using the example of machine learning: "Continued public confidence in the systems that deploy machine learning will be central to its ongoing success, and therefore to realizing the benefits that it promises across sectors and applications" (p. 84).

Trustworthiness

The trustworthiness of AI depends upon its consistency with suitably appearing normative (political and ethical) beliefs and their underlying interests. Ethical guidelines, such as those that the EU Commission has published, represent this approach to trustworthiness very well (European Commission Independent High-Level Expert Group on Artificial Intelligence, 2019). For instance, AI systems should support human autonomy and decision-making, be technically robust and take a preventive approach to risks, ensure prevention of harm to privacy, and be transparent. Also, they should ensure diversity, non-discrimination, fairness, and accountability. These guidelines went into the "ecosystem of trust," a regulatory framework for AI laid down in the European Commission's White Paper on Artificial Intelligence, in which "lack of trust" is "a main factor holding back a broader uptake of AI" (European Commission, 2020, p. 9). Consequently, a "human-centric" approach to the development and use of AI technologies, "the protection of EU values and fundamental rights such as non-discrimination, privacy and data protection, and the sustainable and efficient use of resources are among the key principles that guide the European approach" (European Commission, 2021, p. 31).

In a broader sense, such an approach to trustworthiness applies to any interest groups in politics, economy, and society that express normative beliefs in line with their interests. However, the relevant views are not only those of interest groups but also those among the population of a country, where normative beliefs determine whether a technology like AI appears trustworthy. Ideas of fairness, justice, and transparency are no less relevant for the people than for interest groups. Then, it is less about the technology itself than about the interests that lie behind its applications and their integrity. An important use case is in the labor market, for the (pre)selection of job seekers, described in more detail below.

However, relevant drivers of perceived trustworthiness include not only normative beliefs but also attitudes, expectations, psychological needs, and the hopes and fears relating to AI and robots, in a situation where people lack personal experience with a technology that is still very much in development. In such a situation, trust depends heavily on whether people trust a technology with which they have had no primary experience.

Trust

The ability to develop trust is one of the most important human skills. Self-confidence in one's abilities is certainly a key factor. Trust also plays a paramount role in people's lives in many other respects—for example, from a sociological point of view, as trust in fellow humans, social institutions, and technology. Social systems cannot function without trust that is so functional because it helps people to live and survive, in a world whose complexity always requires more information and skills than any single person can have. I need not be able to build a car to drive it, but I must trust that the engineers designed it correctly. Not everyone is a scientist, but in principle, everyone can develop trust in the expertise of those who have the necessary scientific skills. In everyday life, verifying whether claims correspond to reality is often difficult. Then, the only option is to ask yourself whether you want to believe what you hear and if criteria exist that justify your confidence in their credibility. In short, life in the highly complex modern world does not work without trust. This applies even more to future technologies, such as AI and robots.

Malle and Ullman (2021, p. 4) cite dictionary entries that define "trust" as "firm belief in the reliability, truth, or ability of someone or something"; as "confident expectation of something"; as the "firm belief or confidence in the honesty, integrity, reliability, justice, etc. of another person or thing." In line with these, the authors relate their own concept of trust to persons and agents, "including robots," and postulate that trust's underlying expectation can apply to multiple different properties that the other agent might have. They also postulate that these properties make up four major dimensions of trust: "One can trust someone who is reliable, capable, ethical, and sincere" (Malle & Ullman, 2021, p. 4).

The acceptance of AI and robots requires trust and additional ingredients, a selection of which this chapter highlights. The selection includes the perceived utility and reliability of AI and robots, as well as their closeness to human life. We look at a wider array of areas of application, as well as robotic assistance in the everyday life and care of people. We ask about their respective acceptance, pay special attention to the role that respondents assign to communication in human–robot interaction, and relate this acceptance (i.e., the anticipated willingness to use) to patterns of trust in robotic assistance and autonomous AI, using latent variable analysis. As we detail below, this analysis reveals a pattern that trust in the capability, safeness, and ethical adequacy of AI and robots will build.

Well-Being in Human–Robot Interaction

Trust in AI and robots is one key factor; well-being is a second one. Both prove to be key factors in AI and robots in immediate, everyday human life. People have communication needs that they expect their social interactions to meet. People exchange ideas, take part in different types of conversations, express thoughts and feelings, develop empathy, expect respect and fairness—occasionally also affection and touch—and also react in interpersonal encounters to content, interaction partners, and the course of such encounters with gestures and facial expressions.

Interpersonal interaction can be a very complex structure comprising basic and higher needs, mutual expectations, and verbal and extraverbal stimuli and responses. Complexity is one thing, but social interaction is not only complex. People generally want to feel comfortable in their encounters with other people and find recognition and fairness, and sometimes even more—for example, security. Exceptions prove the rule, but for many people, the search for appreciation and social recognition is recognizable as a basic need. People tend to look for pleasant situations and avoid unpleasant situations as much as possible—at least in general. On the one hand, this describes a situation of interaction between people that can serve as a benchmark for the overwhelmingly difficult task of developing robots that may at least partially substitute for people in such interactions. If people generally expect to have pleasant interpersonal interactions, they will do the same when interacting with robots. On the other hand, this describes a situation highly relevant for attempts to gain acceptance among the population for interactions with robots. This is only possible in the future because people must evaluate such scenarios of human–robot interaction through the emotionally tinted ideas that these scenarios trigger in them today. Since one cannot have acquired any experience with scenarios that do not yet exist, definitions of trust that relate to human–robot interaction cover exactly this uncertainty, as Law and Scheutz (2021, p. 29) put it:

> For example, if persons who have never worked with or programmed a robot before coming in contact with one, they will likely experience a high level of uncertainty about how the interaction will unfold. (...) Therefore, people choosing to work with robots despite these uncertainties display a certain level of trust in the robot. If trust is present, people may be willing to alter their own behavior based on advice or information provided by the robot. For robots who work directly and closely with people, this can be an important aspect of a trusting relationship

The Individual's Self-image

In the present context, we assume that acceptance depends on trust and well-being, and these factors, in turn, on the image of herself that a person possesses. We assume particularly that people who see themselves as open to technical innovation are likely to develop this trust and anticipated well-being, while we expect the opposite from people who rely less on technical innovation and more on the tried and tested. Above all, people who always want to be among the first to try out technical innovations (early adopters) are likely to be open-minded toward AI and interaction with robots, at least substantially more often than others.

We also look at people who orient themselves toward science rather than religion, regarding life issues, a concept that comes from the sociology of religion and refers to a deeper orientation than just a superficial interest in science (Wohlrab-Sahr & Kaden, 2013). We take it up in the context of AI because the very concept of artificial intelligence suggests relating it to the natural intelligence of a person, just to understand what artificial intelligence could mean. Without knowledge of the technical fundamentals of artificial intelligence, such as machine learning, AI can certainly assume a wide variety of meanings, including imaginary content with religious connotations. Accordingly, we assumed that a religiously shaped self-image can go hand-in-hand with a comparatively greater reserve toward AI.

Chapter Overview
This chapter presents findings from the population survey of the Bremen AI Delphi study. The focus is on trust in robotic assistance and willingness to use it, as well as the expected personal well-being in human–robot interaction. Using recent data from Eurostat, the European Social Survey, and the Eurobarometer survey, Chap. 2 extends the analysis to Germany and the EU. We ask if AI could lead to discrimination and whether the state should work as a regulatory agency in this regard. While we confine the exposition to statistical analysis, Chap. 5 discusses in detail the legal challenge of AI. Chapter 2 also investigates the worst-case scenario of cutthroat competition for jobs, using expert ratings from the Delphi. Chapter 3 describes the methodological basis of the study and explains the choice of statistical techniques in this chapter. Two further interfaces merit particular mention. Chapter 4 examines what one can learn from research on robots designed for harsh environments, while Chap. 6 addresses the "communication challenge" of human–robot interaction. Then, Chap. 7 addresses elderly care and the ethical challenges of using assistive robotics in that field.

1.2 Acceptance

1.2.1 Potential for Acceptance Meets Skepticism

In Germany, a high potential for AI acceptance prevails, reflecting an analysis of data from three Eurobarometer studies (European Commission, 2012; European Commission & European Parliament, 2014, 2017). These studies posed questions about the image that people have of robots and AI. Whereas in Germany in 2012, the proportion of those who "all in all" had a "very" or "fairly positive" image of robots was 75%, in 2014, it was 72%. For 2017, the question expanded to include the image of robots and AI, resulting in 64% choosing a "very" or "fairly" positive image in this regard.

A similar picture emerges for our survey in Bremen, where a positive view of robots and artificial intelligence also prevails. A "fairly positive" or "very positive" image of robots and artificial intelligence represent 75% of the responses, and the same proportion (75%) considers robots and artificial intelligence "quite probable" or "quite certain" to be "necessary because they can do work that is too heavy or too dangerous for humans."[1] In addition, 61% consider robots and AI to be "good for society because they help people do their work or do their everyday tasks at home."

---
[1] The figures in this section were presented in a German-speaking public talk held at the University of Bremen in early 2020. See the video at https://ml.zmml.uni-bremen.de/video/5e6a5179d42f1c7b078b4569

The majority even sees the expected consequences of AI for the labor market and one's own workplace as positive rather than negative, as described below. This is in line with the result of an analysis of the comparative perception of 14 risks, which we report in more detail elsewhere (Engel & Dahlhaus, 2022, pp. 353–354). There we asked respondents to rank from a list the five potential risks that worry them most. Respondents hardly regarding "digitization/artificial intelligence" as such a risk (12th place out of 14) is noteworthy; only the specific risk of "abuse/trade of personal data on the Internet" received a top placement in this ranking (fourth place, after "climate change," "political extremism/assaults," and "intolerance/hate on the Internet").

However, at the same time only 33% regard robots and artificial intelligence as "quite probable" or "quite certain" "technologies that are safe for humans." Only 28% view them as "reliable (error-free) technologies," and only 24% as "trustworthy technologies." Other indicators also show this very clearly, especially if specific areas (see below) solicit trust and acceptance. Thus, a high potential for acceptance meets considerable skepticism and a correspondingly wide scope for exploiting this potential.

1.2.2 The Closer to Humans, the Greater the Skepticism toward Robots

In which areas should robots have a role primarily, and in which areas should robots (if possible) have no role? Table 1.1 shows the list that we gave the respondents to answer these two separately asked questions. To rule out question-order effects (the so-called primacy and recency effects), we re-randomized the area sequence for each interview. The ranking asked for places 1 to 5.

When asked about first place, 28% named industry, 16% search and rescue services, 16% space exploration, 10% manufacturing, and 10% marine/deep-sea research. Four of these five areas also shape the preference for second place. There, 26% named marine/deep-sea research, 15% space exploration, 15% industry, 13% health care, and 10% manufacturing. Industry, space exploration, and deep-sea research also dominate the remaining places, followed by manufacturing and health care.

Table 1.1 List of areas where robots should be used primarily vs. not be used at all

List of the areas presented in randomized sequence		
In industry	In caring for people	In the leisure sector
In manufacturing	In education	In transport/logistics
In the service sector	In search and rescue services	In agriculture
In people's private everyday lives	In space exploration	In the military
In health care	In marine/deep-sea research	In no area

Table 1.2 Probabilities of areas where robots should be used primarily vs. not be used at all

Probability that an area is part of the respective TOP 5 ranking set			
Where should robots be used primarily?	Pr (area = element of TOP 5 set)	Where should robots, if possible, not be used at all?	Pr (area = element of TOP 5 set)
... in the industry	0.7546	Care of people	0.6204
... in space exploration	0.7454	people's private lives	0.4954
... in marine/deep-sea research	0.6852	Education	0.4861
... with search and rescue services	0.5139	Military	0.3843
... in health care	0.4306	Leisure sector	0.3704
... in manufacturing	0.3889	Service sector	0.2407
... in transport/logistics	0.3519	Health care	0.1065
... in agriculture	0.1991	Agriculture	0.1065
... at the military	0.1528	No area	0.0880
... in the service sector	0.0972	Transport/logistics	0.0648
... in caring for people	0.0741	Search and rescue services	0.0463
... in people's private everyday lives	0.0694	Manufacturing	0.0231
... in education	0.0463	Industry	0.0093
... in the leisure sector	0.0370	Space exploration	0.0046
... in no area	0.0185	Marine/deep-sea research	0.0

The preferences at the other pole are also noteworthy. When asked where robots should not be in use at all, four areas dominate: caring for people, private everyday life, education, and leisure.

For a more compact picture, we calculated the probability that an area is part of the respective TOP 5 preference set and plotted the two corresponding distributions against each other (Table 1.2 and Fig. 1.1). While industry, space exploration, and marine/deep-sea research are clearly the favorite areas, respondents endorse keeping three areas free of robots: care of people, people's private everyday lives, and education. While these areas polarize responses the most (Fig. 1.1), the following area clusters do the same, though not as dramatically as the former: search and rescue services, health care, manufacturing, and transport/logistics, on the one hand; on the other hand, military, leisure, and service sectors.

For a subset of the areas, an interesting comparison is possible with data for Germany, collected some years ago as part of a Eurobarometer study (European Commission, 2012). Figure 1.2 shows the result of this data analysis. Even if the percentages are not directly comparable across Figs. 1.1 and 1.2 (due to different calculation bases, partly different question wording), the rough pattern relates them to one another and reveals remarkable stability over time. As is true today, the use of

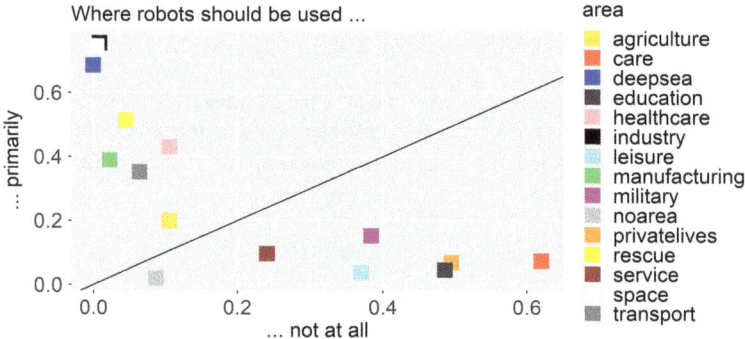

Fig. 1.1 Where robots should be used primarily vs. not be used at all

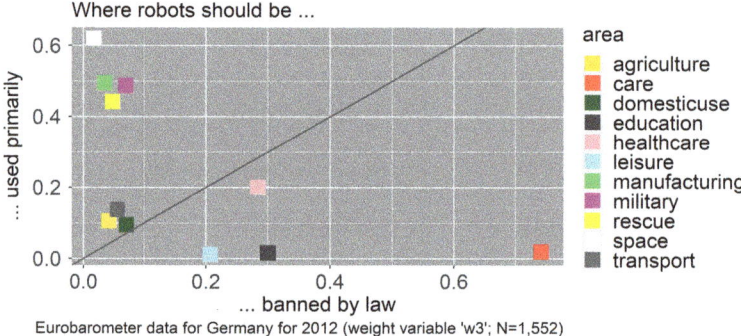

Fig. 1.2 Robotic use: Preferred areas against areas that should be banned by law

robots in space exploration, search and rescue services, and manufacturing had already met with comparatively high levels of acceptance in 2012; the lack of acceptance in care, education, and leisure appears similarly stable. Otherwise, two changes stand out: the use of robots in the military appears more negative today; conversely, their use in health care appears more positive today.

1.2.3 Respondents Find It Particularly Difficult to Imagine Conversations with Robots

We foresee an area comprising two challenges, arising on the premise that assistance robots for the home or for care will only find acceptance in the long term if they can interact with people in a way that people perceive as pleasant communication. We can hardly imagine a human–machine interaction that aligns with repeated frequent encounters but does not satisfy human communication needs. This applies to the extent that humans' inclination toward anthropomorphism assigns assistance robots

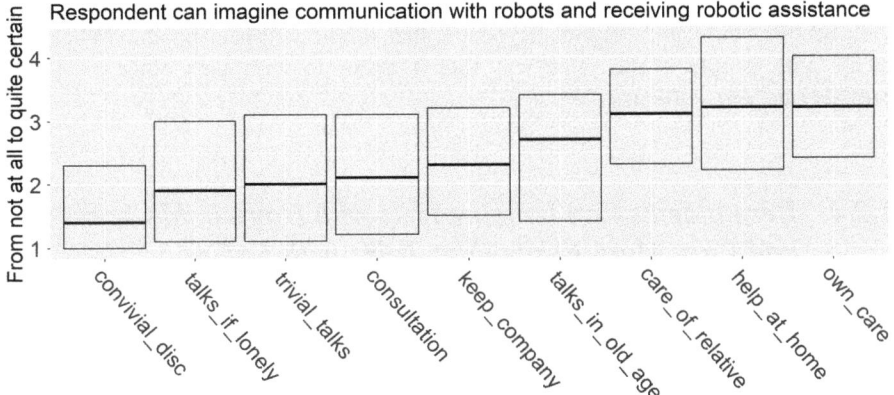

Fig. 1.3 Imagining that humans communicate with robots and receive help from them: Mean values (medians) and pertaining upper/lower bounds of the middle 50% of responses

the role of digital companions in daily interaction (Bovenschulte, 2019; Bartneck et al., 2020). Programming assistant robots with the appropriate communicative skills is the first major challenge; the second lies in the fact that humans still find communicating with a robot extremely difficult to imagine at all. This applies to daily life in general, as Fig. 1.3 and the next paragraph outline, and specifically to robotic assistance in care.

Figure 1.3 displays box plots of the interpolated quartiles (see the appendix, Table 1.7 for the underlying survey-weighted distributions). The introductory question to this block asked if the respondent could imagine conversational situations in which a robot that specializes in conversations would later keep him/her company at home. In Fig. 1.3, this appears in the middle of the chart. The pertaining median of 2.3 indicates a mean value slightly above "probably not," with the middle 50% of responses ranging between 1.5 (this value equals a lower bound exactly in between 1 = "not at all" and 2 = "probably not") and 3.2 (this upper bound lies slightly above the 3 = "possibly" that indicates maximum uncertainty). The respondents consider it unlikely that a robot will keep them company at home in the future. They are even less able to imagine special kinds of conversations—for example, trivial, everyday conversations, in case a respondent feels lonely or ever needs advice on life issues. Respondents nearly completely rule out convivial family discussions in which a robot participates. The same applies to imagining the use of robots that look and move like a pet (Table 1.8). Only conversations in old age with someone no longer mobile were not strictly ruled out, though, in this regard too, the mean value remains slightly below the 3 = "possibly" choice, and the range of the middle 50% of responses includes the 2 = "probably not" and excludes the 4 = "quite probable" at the same time. This is certainly due to the "human factor" in interpersonal communication; humans are humans, robots are machines, no matter how excellent their robotic skills are. Convincing people that robots will later be able to communicate with people in the same way that humans do with each other today will probably be very difficult.

1.2.4 Respondents Can Imagine Help with Household Chores and Care More Easily than Talks with Robots

Can the respondents imagine getting help with household chores? The interview question was: "Research is working on developing robots that will later help people with household chores. We think of examples of this kind: setting and clearing the table, loading and unloading the dishwasher, taking crockery out of cupboards and stowing them back in, fetching and taking away items. For the moment, please imagine that such household robots are already available today: And regardless of financial aspects: Could you imagine receiving help in this way at home?" In Fig. 1.3, the second box plot from the right graphs the pertinent data from Table 1.7: a mean value (median) of 3.2 (slightly above "possibly") and a range from 2.2 to 4.3 that excludes "probably not" and includes "quite probable." Therefore, respondents more easily imagined getting help around the house this way than having conversations with robots.

1.2.5 Robotic Assistance in Care Is as Imaginable as Robotic Assistance with Household Chores

About the same level of acceptance characterizes robotic assistance in care. The survey asked respondents to indicate if they would consent to the involvement of an assistant robot in the care of a close relative and their own care. Two box plots in Fig. 1.3 graph the pertinent data from Table 1.7 in the appendix. The mean values of the two distributions lie slightly above "possibly," with the middle 50% of responses clearly excluding "probably not" and including "quite probable," in the case of respondent's care. Expressed in percentages, this implies that a third of respondents would find "quite probable" or "quite certain" agreeing to the involvement of an assistant robot in the care of a close relative. This proportion increases from 32.4% to 39.1% for the respondent's care (Table 1.3, rows labeled "all").

Twenty-seven percent of the respondents indicated that care is a sensitive issue for them. When asked whether the questions about care "may have been perceived as too personal," 73% answered with "not at all," 19% with "a little bit," 7% with "fairly personal," and 1% with "a lot too personal." Table 1.3 collapses the last three groups and shows for the resulting "sensitive" group how much this group agrees with the participation of a robot in care. Then, only 22.8% would consider "quite

Table 1.3 Consent to robotic assistance in care

Consent to robotic assistance in the care of …							
	If	Not at all	Probably not	Possibly	Quite probable	Quite certain	Don't know
… close relative	All	13.6%	14.1%	36.2%	22.1%	10.3%	3.8%
	Sensitive	5.3%	19.3%	45.6%	19.3%	3.5%	7.0%
… respondent	All	12.9%	12.9%	32.4%	26.7%	12.4%	2.9%
	Sensitive	5.2%	24.1%	36.2%	24.1%	5.2%	5.2%

"Sensitive" if survey questions on care were perceived as too personal. Entries: Row percentages

probable" or "quite certain" the involvement of an assistant robot in the care of a close relative, and only 29.3% would agree to the involvement of an assistant robot in the respondent's care (Table 1.3, rows labeled "sensitive"). Therefore, approval is significantly lower if the topic of "care" is not only of abstract importance. If it is also personally relevant, the approval values drop by almost 10 percentage points.

Irrespective of these results, a little more than half of the respondents expect the involvement of assistance robots in care in the future. In the interview we started the block with questions about care as follows: "The need for care is already a major issue in society, especially for people in need of care and their families themselves. The situation is made even more difficult by a lack of trained specialists. In research, this situation has triggered the development of assistance robots for care. This raises an extremely sensitive question: What would your expectation be: Will it happen within the next ten years that people and robots in care facilities will share the tasks of looking after people in need of care?" Table 1.4 shows that 51.9% expect this.

However, such a development would not meet with unanimous approval. Only about a third of the survey participants would rate this positively. We asked "if robots were used to care for people in need of care," would it be perceived as "very good," "good," "not so good," or "not at all good." Nine percent voted for very good, 26% said it would be good, 37% said it would be not so good, and 23% said it was not at all good (6% did not know).

1.3 Trust in Robotic Assistance and Autonomous AI

Acceptance presupposes trust, and this trust is only available to a limited extent. Figure 1.4 shows this for seven indicators. These concern the use cases "selection of job seekers" (S), "legal advice" (L), "algorithms" (A), and "autonomous driving" (C). Again, the results appear as box plots. We refer to Fig. 1.4 and these indicators in the next sections.

Table 1.4 Expectation that people and robots will share the tasks of care

In future people and robots will share the tasks in care facilities …					
Not at all	Probably not	Possibly	Quite probable	Quite certain	Don't know
4.3%	13.9%	27.9%	42.3%	9.6%	1.9%

1.3.1 Trust in the Integrity of Applicant Selection

To gain trustworthiness, AI as a technology must appear reliable (error-free) and safe for humans. But this is not just about the technology itself. Possible hidden interests on the part of those developing AI or commissioning its development also play a decisive role, so this is also about the interests behind the technology. From a normative (ethical or political) point of view, this is clear, for example, in the recommendations for trustworthy AI, developed for the EU Commission. However, to gain acceptance, AI must also comply with ethical standards from the population's perspective, as clearly appears in the example of applicant selection in the labor market.

We asked the respondents four related questions, starting with: "Please imagine, in large companies, the preselection of applications for vacancies would be carried out automatically by intelligent software. Would you trust that such a preselection would only be based on the applicant's qualifications?" In Fig. 1.4, the second box from left, labeled "S: qualified," describes the responses to this survey question, again in terms of median and upper/lower bound of the interquartile range (also reported in Engel & Dahlhaus, 2022, p. 359, Table 20.A3). This box corresponds to a mean value of 2.6, with the middle 50% of responses ranging between 1.5 and 3.6. Accordingly, the central response tendency is between "probably not" and "possibly," while the middle 50% of the answers include "probably not" and exclude "quite probable."

We relate this trust to the respondent's preference of selection mode and observe the expected close correlation. "Imagine again, in large companies, the preselection under applications for vacancies would be made automatically by intelligent software. What would you personally prefer: automated or human-made preselection?" The percentages in Table 1.9 reveal very clearly that the more the respondents trust that only qualifications count, the more they vote for automated preselection of job applicants and the less they vote for people preselecting.

A related finding is also noteworthy, concerning the two remaining survey questions of the present block. They explore the belief that automated preselection protects applicants from unfair selection. The first was: "Imagine again, in large companies, the preselection under applications for vacancies would be made automatically by intelligent software. Would you trust that such a preselection would effectively protect applicants from unfair selection or discrimination?" In Fig. 1.4, this question is labeled "S: Fair," the left-most box plot. With a mean value of 2.4 and a lower/upper bound of 1.6 and 3.5 of the middle 50% of responses, respondents regard this as just as unlikely as only the applicant's qualification counting. Though

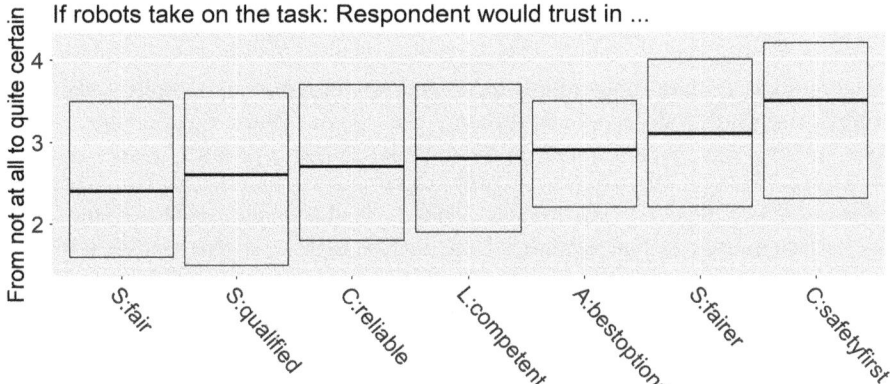

Fig. 1.4 Trust in robotic assistance and autonomous AI: Mean values (medians) and pertaining upper/lower bounds of the middle 50% of responses

the respondents less often prefer automated to human applicant preselection (21% vs. 61.9%; no matter: 11.4%, don't know 5.7%), they consider it possible that automated preselection guards more effectively against discrimination than human preselection. The follow-up question was worded that way: "Imagine again, in large companies, the preselection under applications for vacancies would be made automatically by intelligent software. Would you trust that such a preselection would protect applicants more effectively from unfair selection and discrimination than a human preselection?" In Fig. 1.4, this question is labeled "S: fairer" (the second box plot from the right). Here, we obtain a mean value of 3.1 (slightly above "possibly") and a lower/upper bound of 2.2 and 4.0 of the middle 50% of responses that excludes "probably not" and includes "quite probable."

1.3.2 Legal Advice

AI will likely transform not only simple routine activities but also highly skilled academic professions. Legal advice is just one example. We wanted to know how much people trust legal advice when it is delivered by a robot: "Please imagine that you need legal advice and that you contact a law firm on the Internet. There a robot takes over the initial consultation. Would you trust that it can advise you competently?" In Fig. 1.4, this item is labeled "L: competent." The pertaining quartiles are $Q_1 = 1.9$, $Q_2 = 2.8$, and $Q_3 = 3.7$. They indicate a mean response slightly below "possibly" and a middle range of responses that includes "probably not" but excludes "quite probable."

1.3.3 Algorithms

Relating to algorithms, uncertainty and skepticism also prevail. Despite wide use of comparison portals, do people trust them? We asked: "Please imagine that you are looking for a comparison portal on the Internet to buy a product or service there. Would you trust that the algorithm would show you the best comparison options in each case?" In Fig. 1.4, the item is labeled "A: best options." Here, the major response tendency is "uncertainty" in a double sense: a mean tendency slightly below "possibly," with the middle 50% of responses excluding both "probably not" and "quite probable" ($Q_1 = 2.2$; $Q_2 = 2.9$; $Q_3 = 3.5$).

1.3.4 Self-Driving Cars

The development of autonomous driving is already very advanced, and very likely, self-driving cars will soon be a normal part of the city streetscape. Accidents with such cars during practical tests typically get substantial media attention around the world. That may explain why people are surprisingly still quite skeptical about this technology. We phrased two survey questions that way: "It is expected that self-driving cars will take part in road traffic in the future. Will you be able to trust that the technology is reliable?" In Fig. 1.4, this item is labeled "C: reliable." Here, too, we observe a mean response below "possibly" and lower/upper bounds of the middle 50% of responses that include "probably not" but exclude "quite probable" ($Q_1 = 1.8$; $Q_2 = 2.7$; $Q_3 = 3.7$). At least, the respondents trust in the ethical programming involved, insofar as they trust the "safety first" aspect. In Fig. 1.4, this question is labeled "C: safetyfirst". We asked: "Will you be able to trust that self-driving cars will be programmed to put the safety of road users first?" In this regard, the mean response between "possibly" and "quite probable," with the middle 50% of responses excluding "probably not" and including "quite probable" ($Q_1 = 2.4$; $Q_2 = 3.5$; $Q_3 = 4.2$).

1.3.5 Patterns of Trust and Anticipated Use of Robotic Assistance

Do the indicator variables of trust in robotic assistance and its anticipated use constitute one single basic orientation toward AI and robots that proves invariant across use cases, functions, and contexts? Or should we assume two more or less correlated basic orientations: on the one hand, trust, and on the other, acceptance? Or do people judge this technology in a more differentiated, context-dependent manner, according to the functions and tasks to be fulfilled?

Fig. 1.5 Latent correlations between the factors described in Table 1.5

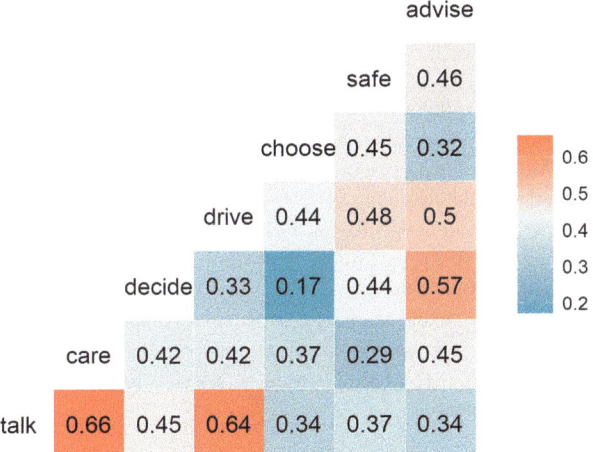

The confirmatory factor analysis (CFA) detailed in the appendix was carried out to answer these questions. It shows that the assumption of a more differentiated structure achieves the best fit of model and data (Table 1.10). Figure 1.5 reports the correlations among the seven factors of trust and anticipated use of robotic assistance that correspond to this latter model. The seven factors involved in this correlation matrix rest on 19 indicator variables, most of which this chapter introduced earlier. The appendix details how these variables constitute the factors in Table 1.11, along with a documentation of question wording and factor loadings.

Respondents who can imagine involving robot assistants in their own care or the care of close relatives can also imagine communicating with robots that specialize in this at home. These ideas are closely related; we observe the relationship at the highest correlation ($r = 0.66$). Conversely, this means that without a willingness to communicate with robot assistants, there is no willingness to involve robots in one's care. Noticeably, *talk* and *drive* also correlate very strongly ($r = 0.64$). Pointedly overstated, anyone who can imagine communicating with a robot at home also has confidence in the technology of self-driving cars, and vice versa. This close relationship between the belief that autonomous driving is reliable and safe for humans and the anticipated readiness to communicate with robots at home might indicate not only the particularly important role of communication in both AI use fields but also the expectation that *assistant* robots at home should be as competent as *autonomously* acting AI.

A third correlation greater than 0.5 concerns *advise* and *decide* ($r = 0.57$); that is, the confidence in competent robotic advice in an important field (e.g., legal advice) and the readiness for getting robotic advice in decision-making. At the same time, *decide* correlates least with *choose* ($r = 0.17$)—that is, the belief that automated preselection would protect job applicants from unfair selection and discrimination. This weak relationship is interesting, insofar as it concerns technology capabilities, on the one hand and, on the other, interests behind special technology applications.

Table 1.5 The seven factors of trust and anticipated use of robotic assistance

Degree of belief ...	
	Trust
Advise	... that a robot would provide competent legal advice
Safe	... that robots and AI are safe for humans, trustworthy, and reliable
Choose	... that an automated preselection of job applicants would protect from unfair selection and discrimination
Drive	... that self-driving cars will be reliable and programmed to put the safety of road users first
	Anticipated use
Decide	... to use an app for smartphones that can advise people making decisions
Care	... to consent to the participation of an assistant robot in one's care
Talk	... to have conversations with specially trained robots and be kept company by them at home

Stated otherwise, highly capable technologies can also be used in the pursuit of interests that people can evaluate quite differently in normative (political and ethical) terms. The perceived performance of a technology is one thing; the perceived integrity of its application is another. Here, both represent widely independent assessment dimensions that require separate consideration.

1.4 Accepting Robotic Assistance and Talking with Robots

In addition to the latent factors and their indicator variables, the present confirmatory factor analysis includes imagining getting help with household chores. This observed variable is regressed on the two latent factors *talk* and *care*. While *talk*'s estimate of effect proves statistically significant:

$$b_{\text{talk}} = 0.657; b/s.e = 5.81; \beta_{\text{talk}} = 0.552.$$

care's estimate of effect approaches such *two*-tailed significance only approximately:

$$b_{\text{care}} = 0.169; b/s.e = 1.76; \beta_{\text{talk}} = 0.166.$$

If this were a *linear* regression, b would indicate the expected change in the target y for a unit change in x_1 (while holding x_2 constant at the same time). However, in the present case, the ordinal scale measures each of the model's *observed* variables (1 = not at all, ..., 5 = quite certain) used throughout this chapter; thus, *probit* regressions estimate all relationships between latent factors and observed variables. Then, the estimates of effect indicate how individuals' values on *talk* and *care* affect *the probability of y falling into specified regions* on the target scale.

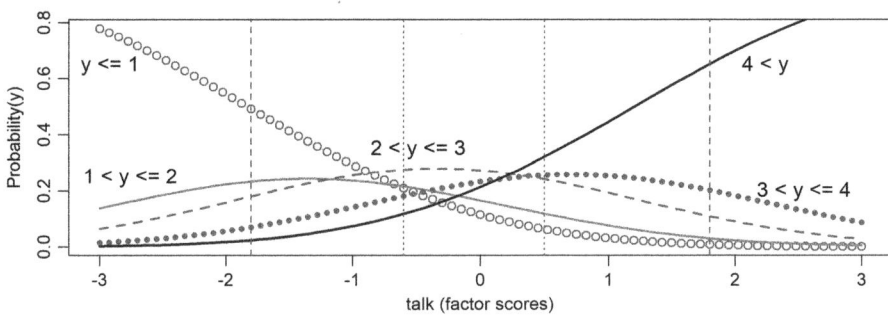

Fig. 1.6 Estimated probabilities of the respondent imagining getting help with household chores as a function of personal acceptance of conversations with appropriately trained assistant robots

Figure 1.6 illustrates this for one of two latent factors, *talk*. In this figure, the outer (dashed) pair of vertical lines indicate the observed minimum and maximum values [−1.8; 1.8] on the latent *talk* scale, while the inner (dotted) pair of vertical lines [−0.6; 0.5] indicate the first and third quartile on this scale of factor scores.

Viewed from left to right, the graphs show the curvilinear course of the probabilities that the answers given on the ordinal y scale are

- less than or equal to 1 ("not at all"),
- in the range of $1 < y \leq 2$ (greater than "not at all," including "probably not"),
- in the range of $2 < y \leq 3$ (greater than "probably not," including "possibly"),
- in the range of $3 < y \leq 4$ (greater than "possibly," including "quite probable"),
- greater than 4 (greater than "quite probable").

With increasing *talk* values (i.e., with stronger beliefs in one's accepting conversations with specially trained robots and being kept company by them at home), the probability curves behave as expected: They fall for "not at all" and they consistently rise for "quite probable." The probabilities between these extremes also develop consistently. In this regard, the graphs in Fig. 1.6 show how the turning point from increasing to decreasing probability values shifts from left to right, depending on whether the probability is considered for smaller or larger values of observed y.

1.5 Technical Innovation, Religion, and Human Values and the Tried and Tested as Elements of the Individual Self-Image

AI and robots represent future technologies. Therefore, assuming that people who are open-minded toward technical innovations will more likely accept them than people who tend to rely on the tried and tested is reasonable. In addition, we assume greater acceptance of robotic assistance among people more oriented toward science than religion, regarding life issues.

The confirmatory factor analysis that Table 1.12 reports is used to compute factor scores on these three dimensions of self-image for each respondent. As expected, the people tend either to be open to technical innovations or to rely on the tried and tested (factor correlation = -0.43). The personal proximity/distance to the market and fashion of technical achievements also plays a role in this contrast.

Conversely, the orientation toward science versus religion in life—as a third dimension—contributes only a partial contrast to the overall picture. On the one hand, this orientation proves to be independent of the openness to technical innovations (0.01^{ns}); on the other hand, it correlates negatively with the orientation toward human values and the tried and tested (-0.39). Regardless of their openness to technical innovations, concerning life issues, people accordingly tend to orient themselves more toward science than human values and religion.

Table 1.6 shows how these dimensions of the individual self-image correlate with the dimensions of trust in AI and robots and their anticipated use. Table 1.6 shows particularly the correlations between the respective scales of factor scores, revealing a clear pattern in this regard. Except for the statistically insignificant relation to *choose*, openness to technical innovation is consistently associated with positive correlations while—again, except for the statistically insignificant relation to *choose* and here also to *safe*—the orientation toward human values and the tried and tested is consistently associated with negative correlations. Therefore, whether someone is open to technical innovations and wants to be among the first to try them out or, on the contrary, relies more on human values and the tried and tested and less on the acquisition of technical achievements, makes a difference.

In terms of statistically significant correlations, the third dimension of self-image is not quite as effective. Those who orient themselves more toward science than religion when it comes to life issues trust competent legal advice by a robot more and would also tend to accept the participation of an assistant robot in one's care. Such an orientation also favors the imagining of feeling comfortable with anticipated situations of human–robot interaction.

Table 1.6 Individual self-image and the anticipated use of/trust in AI. Pearson correlations between factor scores obtained from ordinal probit regression

	Open to technical innovation	Oriented more toward science than religion when it comes to life issues	Relies rather on human values and the tried and tested
Feel good	0.43	0.15	−0.38
Drive	0.42	−0.05	−0.22
Talk	0.39	−0.04	−0.38
Care	0.25	0.26	−0.35
Decide	0.19	0.09	−0.27
Safe	0.18	−0.11	−0.07
Choose	0.13	−0.01	−0.01
Advise	0.16	0.22	−0.33

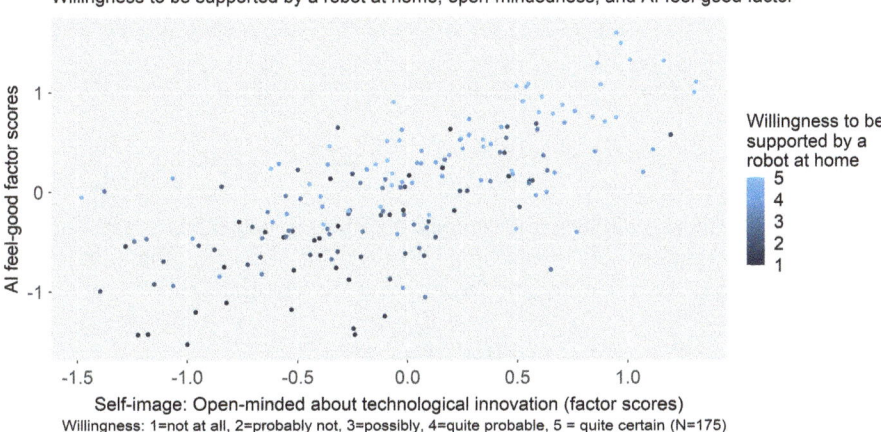

Fig. 1.7 Willingness to be supported by a robot at home, open-mindedness, and AI feel-good factor

1.6 Feeling at Ease with Imagined Situations of Human–Robot Interaction

Whether AI applications will be accepted *for the future* depends crucially on the feelings they trigger in people *today*. Because the applications do not yet exist in peoples' everyday lives, they lack personal experience from which they could form attitudes toward AI and robots. Instead, judgments today depend on people imagining what they may face in this regard in the future. Therefore, we asked the respondents how uncomfortable or comfortable they would feel in eight fictitious situations in which humans interact with robots and, via a confirmatory factor analysis detailed elsewhere. Engel and Dahlhaus (2022, p. 360, Table 20.A4) found that these assessments constitute a single factor. Figure 1.7 plots this feel-good factor against the open-mindedness toward technological innovation. The scattergram also distinguishes the respondents' willingness to get robotic help with household chores, which this chapter describes earlier, and reveals two major relationships: first, the stronger this open-mindedness is, the stronger the feel-good scores are; and second, the higher willingness scores cluster in the upper-right region of the scatterplot and the lower willingness scores in its lower-left region. This expresses all three variables correlating strongly and positively with each other and confirms an equivalent result regarding another target variable, the willingness to seek AI-driven decision support.[2]

We regard the AI feel-good factor as a mechanism by which open-mindedness toward technical innovation leads to anticipated AI use. Formally, it is an *intervening* variable. A simple test can prove if open-mindedness about technological

---

[2] Available at https://github.com/viewsandinsights/AI

innovation, via *this anticipated feeling comfortable with imagined situations of human–robot interaction*, results in the willingness to accept such robotic assistance at home. Regarding the effect of open-mindedness (x) on accepting this assistance (y), a probit regression yields a statistically significant estimate of the effect:

$$b_{yx} = 0.34; b/s.e = 2.65; \beta_{yx} = 0.24; R^2 = 0.059.$$

This direct effect would have to become zero if the feel-good factor were included in the model as a presumably intervening variable. This is exactly what is happening here. If we extend the model by this factor, the direct effect drops to zero

$$b_{yx|z} = -0.01; b/s.e = -0.10.$$

while we observe at the same time two statistically significant estimates of effect, a first (linear regression) effect for the relation of open-mindedness (x) toward feel-good (z)

$$b_{zx} = 0.33; b/s.e = 5.36; \beta_{zx} = 0.43; R^2 = 0.186$$

and a second (probit regression) effect for the relation of feel-good (z) toward acceptance (y)

$$b_{yz} = 1.03; b/s.e = 8.34; \beta_{yz} = 0.56.$$

yielding an explained variance of $R^2 = 0.31$.

1.7 Trustworthiness and Well-Being in the Context of Robotic Assistance

Germans largely have a positive image of artificial intelligence and robots, but they trust this technology to a significantly lower extent. This involves trust in both the technology and the integrity of its applications. The closer AI gets to humans, the more the population questions its acceptance. We observe great acceptance of AI in space exploration and deep-sea research, and at the same time, we observe substantial reservations about its use in people's daily lives. This represents a great challenge for the development of systems of robotic assistance for everyday life and the care of people. However, because large parts of the population have a positive image of AI, there exists a fair potential to convince people (always well-founded) of the trustworthiness of this technology. Following the patterns of trust we describe above, such persuasion campaigns could aim toward specific elements of trust, such as trust in the capability, safety, and ethical adequacy of AI and robotic assistance.

In any case, the further development of AI applications should take people's ideas, needs, hopes, and fears into account. From the analysis above, for example, we can learn that the population is critical of communicating with robots in the domestic context. But we also learn that the readiness to let robots assist in one's care depends largely on this imagined willingness to talk with robots. Furthermore, respondents assign the ability to talk to someone in need of care only a very subordinate role in the qualification profile of a care robot, as Chap. 6 shows.

This requires much persuasion in other respects as well. People judge scenarios of future human–robot interactions based on the emotionally charged ideas that such scenarios trigger in them today. In fact, without primary experience, one can only imagine what such an imaginary situation would be like. The point is just that these beliefs affect the anticipated willingness to use robotic assistance, regardless of how well-founded or unfounded. Therefore, conveying a reliable basis of experience and relying on maximum of transparency in all relevant respects regarding the further development of robotic assistance appear very useful.

Appendix

Table 1.7 Imagination of talking with a robot: interpolated quartiles of survey-weighted frequency distributions

	Q_1	Q_2	Q_3
Each scale: 1 = not at all, 2 = probably not, 3 = possibly, 4 = quite probable, 5 = quite certain			
Could you imagine conversational situations in which a robot that specializes in conversations will later keep you company at home?	1.5	2.3	3.2
What kind of conversations could you imagine?			
Trivial everyday conversations	1.1	2.0	3.1
Conversations in case you ever feel lonely	1.1	1.9	3.0
Conversations in old age, if you are no longer so mobile, can no longer easily socialize with people	1.4	2.7	3.4
In case you should ever need advice on life issues	1.2	2.1	3.1
Convivial discussions with the family, in which a robot also takes part	1.0	1.4	2.3
Could you imagine a robot helping you with household chores?	2.2	3.2	4.3
Consent to the participation of an assistant robot in the care of a close relative	2.3	3.1	3.8
Consent to the involvement of a robot assistant in one's own care	2.4	3.2	4.0

Table 1.8 Robots as pets: Interpolated quartiles of survey-weighted frequency distributions

	Q_1	Q_2	Q_3
Each scale: 1 = not at all, 2 = probably not, 3 = possibly, 4 = quite probable, 5 = quite certain			
Imagine if robots were programmed to keep people company, and robots were made to look and move like a pet, such as a dog or a cat. What do you think about it? Could you imagine keeping a robot as a pet in your home?	1.1	1.7	2.5
Occasionally one hears that for human pets are part of the family as if they were humans themselves. Even if, unlike animals, robots are not living beings, but machines: What would your assumption be, could robots later also fare in the same way as domestic animals do today? So that they too could belong to the family one day?	1.6	2.5	3.4

Table 1.9 Preselection of job applicants and belief that only the qualification counts

Only the applicant's qualification counts	Preference for mode of preselection of job applicants in row percentages				
	Automated	By people	No matter	Don't know	N
Not at all	3.9	90.2	3.9	2.0	51
Probably not	6.0	80.0	4.0	10.0	50
Possibly[a]	30.2	49.1	17.0	3.8	53
Quite probable/certain	41.1	32.1	19.6	7.1	56

[a]Incl. "don't know." A related graph is available at https://github.com/viewsandinsights/AI

Table 1.10 Goodness of fit of three related models of trust and anticipated use of robotic assistance

Model	Robust Chi^2	df	p	CFI	TLI	RMSEA	SRMR
1-factor model: Acceptance and trust collapsed to one factor	887.6	170	0.00	0.82	0.80	0.155	0.178
2-factors model: Acceptance vs. trust	588.98	169	0.00	0.89	0.88	0.119	0.151
7-factor model as reported in Table 1.11 below	164.06	146	0.15	1.0	0.99	0.027	0.049

Table 1.11 Trust in robotic assistance and its anticipated use: CFA factor loadings

	Loadings
Each scale: 1 = not at all, 2 = probably not, 3 = possibly, 4 = quite probable, 5 = quite certain	
HUMAN–ROBOT COMMUNICATION AT HOME	"Talk"
Digital voice assistants are already being used in some private households to answer simple questions to humans. Please imagine if such technical assistants were further developed in such a way that a person can hold conversations with them in the same way that people talk to one another: Could you imagine conversational situations in which a robot that specializes in conversations will later keep you company at home?	0.84
What kind of conversations could you imagine?	
Trivial everyday conversations	0.75
Conversations in case you ever feel lonely	0.93
Conversations in old age, if you are no longer so mobile, can no longer easily socialize with people	0.94
In case you should ever need advice on life issues	0.76
Convivial discussions with the family, in which a robot also takes part	0.75
ASSISTANT ROBOTS IN THE CASE OF NEED FOR CARE	"Care"
Assuming that an assistant robot would—later on—be able to carry out its tasks competently, reliably, and without errors: If you think about your personal environment: Assume that a close relative of yours would need care—And you would be asked for consent to the participation of an assistant robot in the care of this relative. Would you agree?	0.98
Assuming again that an assistant robot would—later on—be able to carry out its tasks competently, reliably, and without errors:	0.97

(continued)

Table 1.11 (continued)

	Loadings
How about yourself: Let us assume that you yourself would one day be in need of care. Would you agree to the involvement of a robot assistant in your own care?	
AI-DRIVEN ADVICE IN THE CASE OF DECISIONS*	"Decide"
What if there were an app for smartphones that can advise people at home or on the go in everyday situations: Would you call in such a personal advisor for decisions that you have to make in everyday life?	0.95
And what if there were an app for smartphones that can advise people in important life situations: Would you call in such a personal advisor for important decisions?	0.92
AUTONOMOUS DRIVING	"Drive"
It is expected that self-driving cars will take part in road traffic in the future. Will you be able to trust that the technology is reliable?	0.88
Will you be able to trust that self-driving cars will be programmed to put the safety of road users first?	0.95
AI PROTECTS AGAINST DISCRIMINATION*	"Choose"
Imagine again, in large companies, the preselection under applications for vacancies would be made automatically by intelligent software. Would you trust that such a preselection would effectively protect applicants from unfair selection or discrimination?	0.91
Imagine again, in large companies, the preselection under applications for vacancies would be made automatically by intelligent software. Would you trust that such a preselection would protect applicants more effectively from unfair selection and discrimination than a human preselection?	0.91
AI IS SAFE FOR HUMANS*	"Safe"
Robots and artificial intelligence are reliable (error-free) technologies	0.75
Robots and artificial intelligence are technologies that are safe for humans.	0.98
Robots and artificial intelligence are trustworthy technologies	0.82
AI ADVISES COMPETENTLY/TRUSTFULLY	"Advise"
Please imagine that you need legal advice and that you contact a law firm on the internet. There a robot takes over the initial consultation. Would you trust that he can advise you competently?	0.88
Please imagine that you are looking for a comparison portal on the internet in order to buy a product or service there. Would you trust that the algorithm would show you the best comparison options in each case?	0.51

$N = 177$. Displayed are standardized factor loadings. All factor loading prove statistically highly significant. The CFA treats all scales as 5 pt ordinal scales using probit regression. Survey weights are employed to handle unit nonresponse. The CFA attains a very acceptable goodness of fit: Robust Chi^2 = 164.06, df = 146, p = 0.15; CFI = 1.0/TLI = 0.99, RMSEA = 0.027; SRMR = 0.049. Because the frequency distributions involve minor percentages of "don't know" responses, these "don't know" responses were recoded to the mid category "possibly," acting on the auxiliary assumption that both categories equivalently express maximal uncertainty. CFA computed using R package "Lavaan." The factors *decide*, *choose*, and *safe* are also part of a similar CFA reported in Engel and Dahlhaus (2022, p. 359)

Table 1.12 Self-image: CFA factor loadings

	Q_1	Q_2	Q_3	
Each item response scale is coded as 1 = not at all, 2 = probably not, 3 = possibly, 4 = quite probable, 5 = quite certain	Interpolated quartiles			Loadings
Would you describe yourself as a person …				
	SELF-IMAGE: OPEN-MINDED*			
… who is open-minded toward technical innovations?	3.5	4.3	4.9	0.88
… who likes to be counted among the first to try out technical innovations?	1.7	2.3	3.5	0.72
… who keeps up with the times?	3.0	3.7	4.3	0.58
SCIENCE vs RELIGION IN PERSONAL LIFE	SCIENCE vs. RELIGION			
… who is more oriented toward science than religion when it comes to personal life issues?	3.4	4.3	4.9	0.80
… who is religious?	1.1	1.8	3.2	−0.64
	HUMAN VALUES AND THE TRIED AND TESTED			
… who relies on the tried and tested first and foremost?	2.7	3.4	4.2	0.70
… who does not have to go along every fashion?	3.7	4.3	4.9	0.38
… for whom life is first and foremost about human values, not technical achievements?	4.0	4.7	5.1	0.59

$N = 189$. Displayed are standardized factor loadings. The CFA treats all scales as 5 pt ordinal scales using probit regression. Survey weights are employed to handle unit nonresponse (GOF: Robust Chi^2 = 39.20, df = 15, p = 0.001; CFI = 0.91/TLI = 0.84, RMSEA = 0.093; SRMR = 0.090). The computation of interpolated quartiles is based on weighted frequency distributions too. Because the frequency distributions involve minor percentages of "don't know" responses, these "don't know" responses were recoded to the mid category "possibly," acting on the auxiliary assumption that both categories equivalently express maximal uncertainty. R packages used in this analysis: "Survey," "Lavaan." The factor *open-minded* is also part of a similar CFA reported in Engel and Dahlhaus (2022, p. 359)

References

Bartneck, C., Belpaeme, T., Eyssel, F., Kanda, T., Keijsers, M., & Sabanovic, S. (2020). *Human-robot interaction: An introduction*. Cambridge University Press.

Bovenschulte, M. (2019). *Digitale Lebensgefährten – der Anthropomorphismus sozialer Beziehungen [Digital companions - the anthropomorphism of social relationships]*. Büro für Technikfolgenabschätzung beim Deutschen Bundestag (TAB). Themenkurzprofil Nr. 31. Retrieved December 28, 2021, from https://doi.org/10.5445/IR/1000133933

Engel, U., & Dahlhaus, L. (2022). Data quality and privacy concerns in digital trace data. In U. Engel, A. Quan-Haase, S. Liu, & L. Lyberg (Eds.), *Handbook of computational social science, Vol. 1 - Theory, case studies and ethics* (pp. 343–362). Routledge. https://doi.org/10.4324/9781003024583-23

European Commission. (2012, February–March). *Brussels: Eurobarometer 77.1. TNS OPINION & SOCIAL, Brussels [Producer]*. GESIS, Cologne [Publisher]: ZA5597, dataset version 3.0.0, 2014. Retrieved from https://doi.org/10.4232/1.12014

European Commission. (2020). *White paper on artificial intelligence – A European approach to excellence and trust*. Retrieved December 28, 2021, from https://ec.europa.eu/info/sites/default/files/commission-white-paper-artificial-intelligence-feb2020_en.pdf

European Commission. (2021). *Annexes to the Communication from the Commission to the European Parliament, the European Council, the Council, the European Economic and Social Committee and the Committee of the Regions. Fostering a European approach to Artificial Intelligence*. Retrieved December 28, 2021, from https://op.europa.eu/en/publication-detail/-/publication/01ff45fa-a375-11eb-9585-01aa75ed71a1/language-en

European Commission & European Parliament. (2014, November–December). *Brussels: Eurobarometer 82.4. TNS opinion, Brussels [Producer]*. GESIS, Cologne [Publisher]: ZA5933, dataset version 6.0.0, 2018. Retrieved from https://doi.org/10.4232/1.13044

European Commission & European Parliament. (2017, March). *Brussels: Eurobarometer 87.1. TNS opinion, Brussels [Producer]*. GESIS, Cologne [Publisher]: ZA6861, data set version 1.2.0. Retrieved from https://doi.org/10.4232/1.12922

European Commission Independent High-Level Expert Group on Artificial Intelligence. (2019). *Ethics guidelines for trustworthy AI*. Retrieved December 28, 2021, from https://ec.europa.eu/futurium/en/ai-alliance-consultation.1.html

Law, T., & Scheutz, M. (2021). Trust: Recent concepts and evaluations in human-robot interaction. In C. S. Nam & J. B. Lyons (Eds.), *Trust in human-robot interaction* (pp. 27–57). Academic Press. https://doi.org/10.1016/B978-0-12-819472-0.00002-2

Malle, B. F., & Ullman, D. (2021). A multidimensional conception and measure of human-robot trust. In C. S. Nam & J. B. Lyons (Eds.), *Trust in human-robot interaction* (pp. 3–25). Academic Press. https://doi.org/10.1016/B978-0-12-819472-0.00001-0

The Royal Society. (2017). *Machine learning: The power and promise of computers that learn by example*. Retrieved December 28, 2021, from https://royalsociety.org/~/media/policy/projects/machine-learning/publications/machine-learning-report.pdf

Wohlrab-Sahr, M., & Kaden, T. (2013). Struktur und Identität des Nicht-Religiösen: Relationen und soziale Normierungen [Structure and identity of the non-religious: Relations and societal norms]. *Kölner Zeitschrift für Soziologie und Sozialpsychologie, 65*, 183–209. https://doi.org/10.1007/s11577-013-0223-8

Michael Beetz is a professor for Computer Science at the Faculty for Mathematics & Informatics of the University Bremen and a head of the Institute for Artificial Intelligence (IAI). IAI investigates AI-based control methods for robotic agents, with a focus on human-scale everyday manipulation tasks. He is the coordinator of the German Collaborative Research Centre EASE (Everyday Activity Science and Engineering). His research interests include plan-based control of robotic agents, knowledge processing and representation for robots, integrated robot learning, and cognitive perception.

Uwe Engel is a Professor at the University of Bremen (Germany), where he held a chair in sociology from 2000 until his retirement in autumn 2020. In 2007, he founded the Social Science Methods Centre of Bremen University, and directed this institution until 2020. Current work focuses on computational social science and human–robot interaction. See https://www.viewsandinsights.com/en/welcome-to-views-insights and https://orcid.org/0000-0001-8420-9677 for details.

Nina Hoyer studied biology at the University of Oldenburg. In 2016, she completed her Dr. rer. nat. in the field of neurobiology at the Center for Molecular Neurobiology, Hamburg (ZMNH). Since 2017, she started a position as a research associate at the Robotics Innovation Center at the German Research Center for Artificial Intelligence GmbH in Bremen, followed by research position at the Research Group Robotics of the University of Bremen. Her work focusses on the coordination and acquisition of projects.

Lorenz Kähler, born in 1973, studied law and philosophy in Heidelberg, London, and Göttingen. Ph.D. in law about overruling decisions in 2003; habilitation about the justification and concept of default rules 2010, Ph.D. in philosophy about duties to oneself in 2021. Since 2011, Professor for Private Law, Civil Procedure, and Legal Philosophy at the University of Bremen. Main research area: contract theory and the social ontology of law.

Hagen Langer is a senior researcher at the Institute for Artificial Intelligence at the University of Bremen. His research interests include natural language processing, knowledge representation, multiagent systems, cognitive robotics, and machine learning. He received a doctoral degree from Georg-August-Universität Göttingen and he also holds a habilitation from the University of Osnabrück. Since 2017, he is the managing director of the Collaborative Research Center EASE—Everyday Activity Science and Engineering (http://www.ease-crc.org).

Holger Schultheis holds a Diploma in Computer Science and in Psychology from Saarland University (2004). He received his Ph.D. (2009) and habilitation (2017) in Computer Science from the University of Bremen, where he is currently a senior lecturer. He also works as a consultant and project manager for AI and Data Science at neusta analytics & insights GmbH. By combining insights from cognitive science and methods from artificial intelligence, he works toward understanding, improving, and controlling complex human–machine collaborative systems. In doing so, one focus is on creating sustainable and user-friendly technical systems that operate with high resource efficiency.

Sirko Straube studied neurobiology and computer science at the Albert-Ludwigs-University Freiburg, Germany, where he graduated in 2005. After completing his dissertation about human object recognition in 2009, he joined the Robotics Innovation Center in Bremen, Germany, first at the University Bremen—later at DFKI GmbH, leading projects focused on human–machine interaction, machine learning, hybrid teams of humans and robots, and advanced training for companies. Since 2015, Sirko Straube is the institutes deputy head. His core interests are in cooperation of industry and research, the successful knowledge transfer, and to bring more transparency about current AI-trends into the public awareness.

Open Access This chapter is licensed under the terms of the Creative Commons Attribution 4.0 International License (http://creativecommons.org/licenses/by/4.0/), which permits use, sharing, adaptation, distribution and reproduction in any medium or format, as long as you give appropriate credit to the original author(s) and the source, provide a link to the Creative Commons license and indicate if changes were made.

The images or other third party material in this chapter are included in the chapter's Creative Commons license, unless indicated otherwise in a credit line to the material. If material is not included in the chapter's Creative Commons license and your intended use is not permitted by statutory regulation or exceeds the permitted use, you will need to obtain permission directly from the copyright holder.

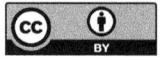

Chapter 2
Artificial Intelligence and the Labor Market: Expected Development and Ethical Concerns in the German and European Context

Uwe Engel and Lena Dahlhaus

Abstract The chapter examines the question of whether people must fear for their jobs due to artificial intelligence (AI). A "competitive scenario" with a design to test for this appeared in the Delphi survey. The chapter shows how realistic this scenario is and its sociological implications, with a basis in expert opinions. In addition, the chapter sheds light on how much people see AI affecting themselves in their jobs, their future standard of living, and quality of life. The results in these respects paint a much more positive picture than the public discussion of AI leads us to expect. The chapter deals with ethical concerns that AI could lead to discrimination in the labor market and the perceived need for public policy interventions to ensure that AI develops ethically. An aggregate data analysis reveals substantial variations across EU countries and significant correlations with a country's prosperity, risk of poverty, multi-ethnicity, and inherent trust in institutions and fellow men. We examine the odds of such concerns in Germany, as a function of socio-structural variables.

Keywords Artificial intelligence · Labor market · Ethical concerns · Public policy · Regulation

2.1 Introduction

Artificial intelligence, robotics, and their joint potential to influence the future labor market have been under labor-market researchers' scrutiny for some time. Their influence and closely related technologies, such as machine learning, have already shown great potential as drivers of economic growth (Graetz & Michaels, 2015;

U. Engel (✉)
University of Bremen, Bremen, Germany
e-mail: uengel@uni-bremen.de

L. Dahlhaus
University of Oldenburg, Oldenburg, Germany
e-mail: lena.dahlhaus@uol.de

Aghion et al., 2019), and their influence is likely to accelerate in the future. Beginning with industrialization, the influence of automation on work has been a continuous presence, igniting both beneficial economic growth and structural changes concerning the labor market. Critical views concerning its influence on human labor conditions have appeared for just as long. Already in 1930, economist John M. Keynes had put his economic pessimism stemming from technological advancement into words, proposing:

> We are being afflicted with a new disease of which some readers may not yet have heard the name, but of which they will hear a great deal in the years to come—namely, *technological unemployment.* This means unemployment due to our discovery of means of economising the use of labour outrunning the pace at which we can find new uses for labour. (Keynes, 1930/2010)

AI will change the working and professional world and, thus, a central pillar of life in society. In the past, human–robot collaboration and the use of AI was primarily limited to the takeover of repetitive tasks in the industrial workplace setting, but it has increasingly entered new fields—for example, the fields of customer service and health care (Decker et al., 2017; Huang & Rust, 2018). Jobs formerly deemed not substitutable through robots are no longer so to the same extent, raising fears of mass unemployment (Frank et al., 2019; Webb, 2019). However, research rates how much AI-driven automation threatens jobs differently because the labor market is complex, and the speed of technological progress is difficult to estimate.

Such expectations include major changes in company business models: the automation of routine processes and AI enhancement and support of a large part of the tasks awaiting solution. Thus, AI will become a constant companion of people in the workplace. According to Eurobarometer data for 2017 (European Commission & European Parliament, 2017), to a remarkable extent, working people attribute to AI the potential to take over their jobs in the future. Only 59% completely rule this out for themselves, women at a higher proportion than men (66–52%). However, AI will not only cost jobs; it will also create new ones. Also, AI may just lead to changed employee qualification requirements (Lane & Saint-Martin, 2021).

Still, 3 years ago, the expectation was that one in four employees in Germany would have to anticipate AI replacing their job, and that trend is rising.[1] According to this IAB study, manufacturing professions, company-related service professions, professions in corporate management and organization, transport, and logistics professions, as well as commercial professions would be among the most affected. Meanwhile, a more recent IAB study assumes for Germany that 34% of jobs are subject to high substitution potential. In addition, the study indicates a substantial increase in this figure from 15% in 2013 to 34% in 2019 (Wrobel & Althoff, 2021).

Workers must adapt and develop new skills to stay competitive in changing areas of work. At present, the consensus in labor-market research states that human–

---

[1] Along with a selection of its findings, a report about this IAB study appears in an article published on 16 February 2018 at https://www.welt.de/wirtschaft/article173642209/Jobverlust-Diese-Jobs-werden-als-erstes-durch-Roboter-ersetzt.html

machine coexistence will be the future norm (Hamid et al., 2017; Bankins & Formosa, 2020).

AI touches not only simple routine activities. It is also advancing into areas of high-quality academic work. Predictably, recommendations and decisions will be more automatic in the future. "The McKinsey Global Institute estimates that through highly developed algorithms and thinking machines alone, worldwide 140 million knowledge workers will be replaced by technology in the coming years" (Goffart, 2019, p. 58). In fact, white-collar jobs are at risk, even in most creative areas like music and painting (Ford, 2016, pp. 113–114).

Similarly, Baldwin (2019, pp. 4–5) refers to skills that computers never had before—"things like reading, writing, speaking, and recognizing subtle patterns"—making "white-collar robots" fierce competitors for office jobs. He even talks of "globotics," a combination of a new form of globalization and a new form of robotics, which he sees as different from the "century-old stories" of automation and globalization, "coming inhumanly fast, and it will seem unbelievably unfair."

Regarding robots in the future taking over automatable activities, any associated job losses will threaten the professional existence of many people and families. Even if, in the next few years and decades, AI will create new jobs to the same extent—perhaps even more jobs than will be lost—the question remains whether these jobs will also offer the same economic and social security. Quite conceivably, AI will act as a catalyst for the erosion of standard employment. Digital crowd-working platforms, for example, can certainly be harbingers of a reality in which the model of "permanent employment with social security" as the livelihood of the middle class will have substantially lost its importance. In the platform economy already, only a few permanent employees with gigantic sales and value constitute such companies. At the same time, attention is turning to the fact that the design of business models aims at shifting the business risk from the platform to the respective users (Adams-Prassl, 2019).

As a consequence of technological advancement in artificial intelligence and robotics today, new challenges and possibilities concerning the structure and organization of work are continuously emerging and may certainly lead to future societal changes on a larger scale. With artificial intelligence evolving rapidly, the effort toward measuring and understanding the impact of such changes is of particular importance for social science research. While discussed extensively, empirical evidence detailing the extent of expected human job replacement is comparatively little, in addition to yielding different outcomes altogether (Felten et al., 2018).

Research that aims at predicting future events as complex as labor-market changes is a challenging endeavor. An important pillar in assessing future characteristics of a labor market that automation shapes even more is the gathering of expert knowledge. As Chap. 3 details, for such an assessment we used a real-time Delphi design that confronts the experts with a series of scenarios of different complexity. One of these scenarios is the "competitive scenario," (see Sect. 2.1.), with a related population view (see Sect. 2.2). Following this, we devote Sect. 2.3 to ethical concerns that AI could lead to discrimination in the labor market and beyond. No doubt, biases in human perception can and do lead to discriminatory practices

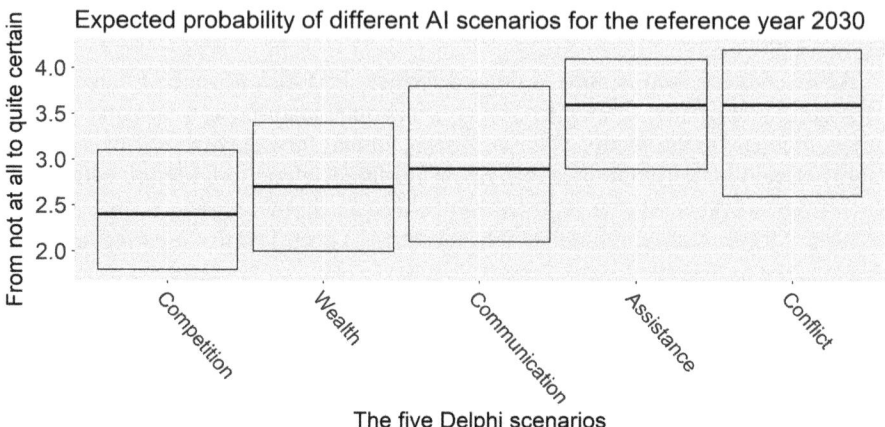

Fig. 2.1 The five scenarios the Delphi study posits

(e.g., toward job applicants), but letting algorithms aid in the process raises concerns that may not be unfounded, given the evidence of previous occurrences of systematic discrimination in automated decision-making (Kleinberg et al., 2020; Ferrer et al., 2021). In this regard as well, findings from the Delphi appear below. However, the major focus of Sect. 2.3 is the analysis of European countries, using data from Eurostat and aggregated survey data from Eurobarometer 92.3 and the European Social Survey. Section 2.3 also presents an analysis of the social structure of ethical concern that AI could lead to discrimination.

2.2 AI and the Labor Market

2.2.1 The Competitive Delphi Scenario: Expert Views

The competitive scenario is one out of five scenarios the Delphi survey poses. The Delphi reveals destructive competition for permanent appointments as an unlikely worst-case scenario (Fig. 2.1) that depicts a situation affecting even the highly skilled middle class. It describes a job market where AI handles a steadily increasing part of even highly skilled routine jobs. This trend accompanies declining workforce demand, forcing people into precarious employment on digital crowd-working platforms and threatening even the stability of democracy.

Engel and Dahlhaus (2022, p. 345) state that

> though AI is expected to shape the job market in general, highly qualified staff is regarded as not that concerned, at least not for the near future. While 38 percent of the Delphi respondents anticipate a clear reduction of permanent appointments due to AI in Germany in 2030, the survey's reference year, only 20 percent believe in corresponding job losses for

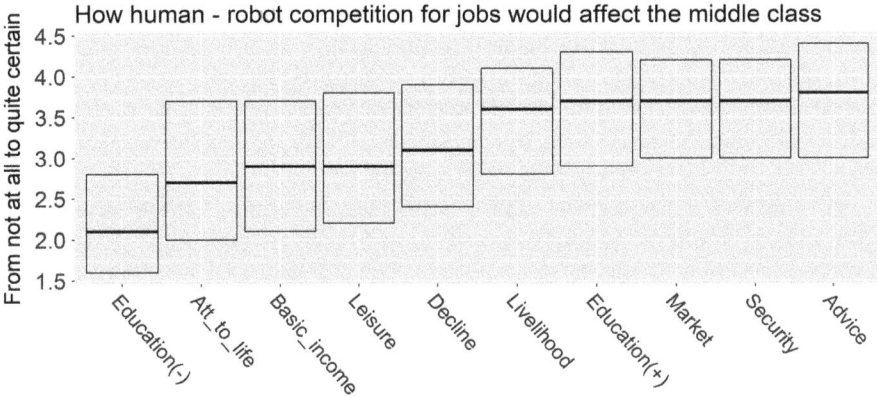

Fig. 2.2 How human–robot competition for jobs would affect the middle class

highly skilled academic personnel. In this respect, the prevailing expert opinion (78 percent) anticipates primarily changing job specifications due to AI.

The fact that the substitution potential of jobs for highly qualified people is comparatively lower aligns with the recent IAB study cited above. However, a residual uncertainty may still exist. Even if AI cannot easily replace jobs that require demanding academic qualifications, the question remains whether the current assumption that these qualifications will protect them effectively against substitution is valid, especially against the background that the technology is still developing. In any case, the Delphi participants currently assume a rather low risk, partly concerning their own job profile. University education is an apt example. Using the standard response scale that appears throughout the surveys of the Bremen AI Delphi study ($Q_1 = 1.6$; $Q_2 = 2.1$; $Q_3 = 2.8$), the respondents rate the following situation as unlikely to occur: "AI has changed academic teaching in the country. In many bachelor-degree programs, robot assistants now take over the lecture-accompanying exercises and exam preparation for students."

The Delphi reveals the scenario of a destructive human–robot competition for permanent appointments as an unlikely worst-case scenario. *But what if not?* That competitive scenario would hit the well-educated middle class particularly hard. Granted, the intensified competition in the labor market would effectively turn out as this scenario assumes. Then, what are the expected consequences for the reference year 2030? Figure 2.2 displays the subjective expectations of some such consequences, four of which would appear likely: increased importance of education as a key to professional success, the demand for a lifelong and comprehensive tax-financed protection of an acceptable livelihood, accompanied by a controversial public discussion of a corresponding restructuring of the taxes and social security contribution system; a weakening of the liberal center in favor of the fringes of the political spectrum; and greater demand for psychosocial counseling.

The scales above include the following observations. For the reference year 2030, the "attitude to life" scale describes a situation that appears *rather unlikely than likely* to the Delphi respondents: "People's attitude towards life will not have changed significantly." On the one hand, the middle 50% of responses include "probably not" and, on the other hand, exclude "quite probable," with the median located slightly below "possibly," expressing maximum uncertainty.

Three further consequences appear essentially *uncertain*, exhibiting a narrow dispersion of responses around "possibly" while the middle 50% of responses exclude both bounds, "probably not and "quite probable." They are: "Since the state has guaranteed every citizen a basic income since 2025, AI has been viewed largely positively by the population—despite all competition" (Basic_income); "People would have to spend much more time than before to secure their living standard; time that is missing for a meaningful way of life" (Leisure); "An attitude towards life characterized by deep insecurity and fears of social decline will have spread across the population" (Decline).

Finally, a group of statements describes consequences that appear *rather likely than unlikely* to the Delphi respondents. Here, the middle 50% of responses exclude "probably not" and include "quite probable." One is the statement that in the meantime, the population has massively asked the state for a comprehensive and lifelong tax-financed safeguarding of an acceptable standard of living (Livelihood). It also applies to the expected public debate on this topic. We phrased a corresponding statement as: "The decline in the factors of production of labor and human capital in value added, which was forecast in the decade before last, has meanwhile come true. Since then, a fundamental restructuring of the system of taxes and social security taxes has been the subject of very controversial public debate" (Security). Third is the statement concerning the central role of education, which the responses to two opposing statements indicate. On the one hand, we observe a clear rejection of the statement that for many, education is no longer the key to professional success. The people ask themselves: "Why invest in education if it doesn't pay off for me?" (Education $(-)$). On the other hand, the Delphi respondents found it much more likely to expect that many consider education to be "the" key to professional success. Again for the reference year 2030, they expect that in recent years, Germany will have seen a real run to the qualification offers of universities and institutions of further education and training (Education $(+)$). Furthermore, it is more likely than unlikely that confidence in the free market would decline; the liberal center would have lost much popularity, while the fringes of the political spectrum would have gained significantly (Market). And people would have to pay a price for the burdens of increased competition. In the year 2030, the more likely consequences would also include a sharp rise in recent years in the demand for psychological and pastoral advice (Advice).

2.2.2 AI and the Anticipated Standard of Living and Quality of Life: Population Views

We balanced the wording of our survey question as well as possible:

> It is widely expected that the introduction of artificial intelligence techniques will have an impact on the labor market. Three possibilities are foreseen: Downsizing: companies will reduce the number of their permanent employees; Compensation: job losses will be offset by job gains; Gain: More new jobs will be created than old ones will be eliminated. What do you suspect: What will the labor market likely to come to in the next ten years?

Even if only 7% expect a gain and 56% expect downsizing (compensation: 35%; don't know: 3%), the answers to the following question clearly indicate anticipation of only a limited personal concern if just 6% expect substantial replacement. "If you are currently employed, do you think that your current job could be taken over by a robot or artificial intelligence in the future?" "Yes, completely" [1%]; "yes, for the most part" [5%]; "yes, but only partly" [41%]; "no, not at all" [51%]; "don't know" [2%]. This is likely to be the case, although only around half of the respondents assume that robots cannot replace them at all on the job, at least if one also considers the perceived impact on one's living standard and quality of life. In this regard, significantly greater proportions of people expect positive rather than negative effects for themselves. The survey question was: "What would you guess: Will artificial intelligence change the economy and the labor market in the country in such a way that these changes will have a positive or negative effect on your future standard of living? Or do you not expect any impact in this regard?" Thirty-five percent expected positive impact, 27% no impact, and 19% negative impact (don't know: 19%). Even more pronounced is the apparent imbalance in the case of one's quality of life. "Just as artificial intelligence may affect jobs and a person's standard of living; this technology may also affect a person's quality of life in a broader sense. (...) What would you guess? Could robots and artificial intelligence be something that has a positive or negative impact on your quality of life? Or would you not expect any effects in this regard?" Here, 46% expected positive impact, 26% no impact, and 13% negative impact (don't know: 16%). A case study in Italy reports a similarly positive expectation (Operto, 2019, p. 291).

2.2.3 Ethical Concerns

AI applications that are error-free and safe for humans are not enough to consider them trustworthy in society. These properties are certainly necessary but not sufficient. The same applies to the usefulness of AI applications since usefulness or functionality alone cannot guarantee sufficient social acceptance. Achieving trustworthiness can only occur with adherence to ethical standards at the same time, in the population and among social stakeholders, both of whom "trustworthy AI" must convince to gain sufficient social acceptance.

Using the labor market and job search as an example can easily demonstrate the fact that this ethical dimension can quickly gain personal relevance in everyday life. In Chap. 1, we raised the question of the integrity of an AI-supported preselection of applicants for vacancies in large companies. While the analysis there is based on the population survey that we carried out for Bremen at the end of 2019, this section aims to extend the perspective to the European level. With Eurobarometer 92.3 (European Commission, 2019), a population survey is available that was fielded at the same time that we conducted the survey in Bremen.[2] The Eurobarometer involves a few AI-related survey questions, two of which the present section takes up.

2.2.3.1 Regulation Mode and Trust in Institutions

As part of our Delphi, we asked the respondents from science and politics to assess a scenario for the reference year 2030 that Chap. 5 of this volume also addresses:

> Since its introduction in 2019, the implementation of the EU Commission's ethics guideline for trustworthy AI has preoccupied the political discussion and the courts in the country. The focus is on the dispute about the guarantee of people's right to self-determination and the protection against discrimination, stigmatization, and violation of personal rights through AI systems. Also in focus: questions of liability for self-learning, autonomously acting AI systems, their ethically acceptable programming and the question of what rights robots should be granted who live with people in common households. What would your expectation be: will this scenario become a reality?

Using the standard response scale implemented throughout the surveys of the present study, respondents rated this scenario as likely rather than unlikely ($Q_1 = 2.6$; $Q_2 = 3.6$; $Q_3 = 4.2$). This is the scenario labeled "Conflict" in Fig. 2.1. In the present context, three single follow-up ratings are worth mentioning. Viewed from the reference year 2030 again, the first of these ratings addressed the premise that the EU ethics guideline had been a legal requirement for universal compliance since 2025: "The AI assistance systems developed for recruitment of job seekers have since then to be officially approved to guarantee protection against discrimination, stigmatization, and violation of personal rights." The respondents rated this scenario as possible to quite probable.

In the present context, both the assumed need for state regulation and the problem of discrimination itself are important. For instance, as part of Eurobarometer 92.3, the survey asked the European population about the need for public policy intervention, if industry providers of Artificial Intelligence can deal with these issues themselves, or no need of specific action to ensure that the development of Artificial Intelligence applications occurs in an ethical manner (survey question QF4).

---

[2]Eurobarometer 92.3 (GESIS Study number ZA7601), fieldwork between Mid-November to Mid-December 2019.

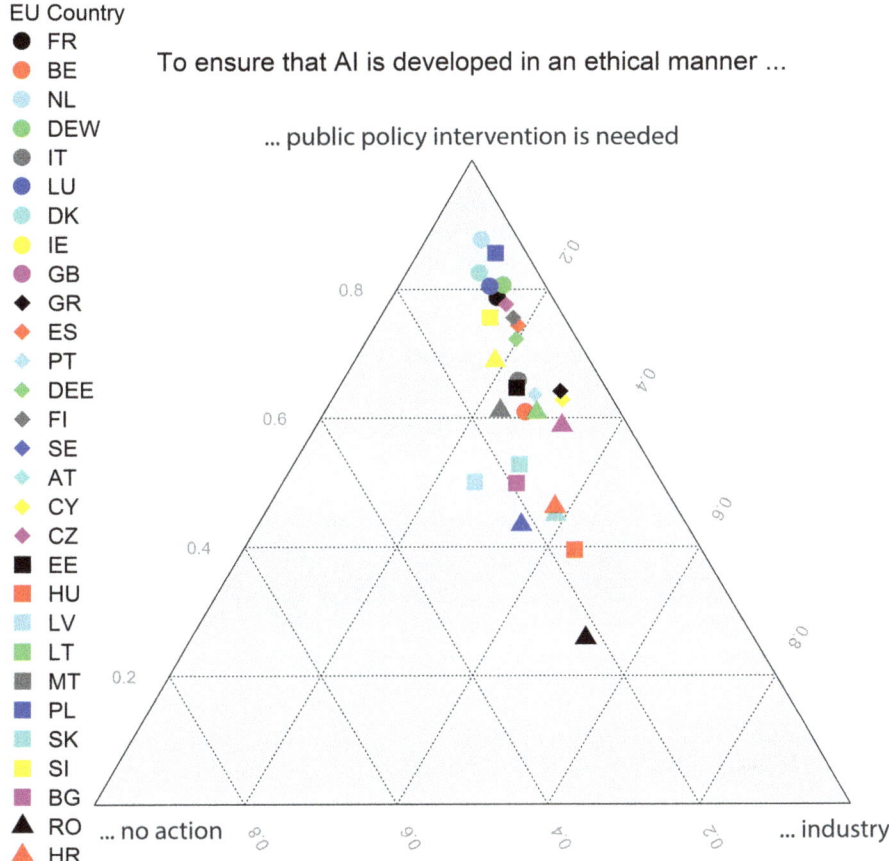

Fig. 2.3 Regulation mode to ensure that AI is developed in an ethical manner

Figure 2.3 graphs the weighted country-specific frequency distributions, and Table 2.3 documents them in the appendix to this chapter.

The graph localizes each country using its three proportions for "public policy intervention is needed" (Axis runs from bottom left [0] to top [1.0]); "industry providers of Artificial Intelligence can deal with these issues themselves" (Axis runs from top [0] to bottom right [1.0]); and "no specific action is needed" (Axis runs from bottom right [0] to bottom left [1.0]). By and large, the resulting spread indicates this situation: (1) There exists a clear tendency toward preferring public policy intervention over self-regulation by the relevant industry. (2) There exists a considerable spread between the poles of "public policy" and "industry," with, at the same time, (3) significantly less between-country variation in the preference for "no specific action is needed." Thus, for the most part, a propagated need appears for state or industry regulation. All of this, at least by and large, is because the scatter plot in Fig. 2.3 and the frequency distributions in Table 2.3 show that pronounced differences in the numbers between the countries exist at the same time.

Table 2.1 (first outcome row) also indicates this spread in the preference for public policy intervention. If we compute for each country the percentage of respondents who express this preference (using the weighted frequency distributions), we obtain one such value for each country. Thus, 28 countries yield 28 corresponding percentages, and Table 2.1 displays the summary statistics of the aggregate variable that these 28 values constitute. Such variables now characterize the countries, not the people living in them (aggregate data analysis). For instance, Table 2.1 shows that the lowest observed percentage of people expressing said preference is 19.0, and Table 2.3 in the appendix to this chapter reveals that this value pertains to Romania. At the other pole, Table 2.1 indicates a maximum value of 77.5 percentage points, while Table 2.3 reveals that this value pertains to the Netherlands. All other countries range between these min/max boundaries and

Table 2.1 Country-level summary statistics and correlations[a]

	Concern[b]	Public policy intervention[b]	Summary statistics (country level)				
	Correlations (country level)			Quartiles			
			Min	Q_1	Q_2	Q_3	Max
Public policy intervention[b]			19.0	33.6	48.5	56.7	77.5
Concern[b]		0.78	16.6	27.4	34.2	38.6	57.1
			PROSPERITY & POVERTY				
Living standards: Gross domestic product (GDP per capita in PPS)[c]	0.50	0.52	51.0	71.0	91.5	118.5	261.0
Poverty risk[c]	−0.38	−0.34	12.5	17.2	20.1	24.8	32.8
Deprivation[c]	−0.34	−0.39	5.0	7.4	12.6	17.1	32.6
Income deprivation[d]	−0.48	−0.53	6.7	14.1	22.2	28.6	67.0
			MULTI-ETHNICITY				
RH-Ethnicity[d]	0.30	0.26	0.0	0.04	0.15	0.21	0.24
RHF-Ethnicity[d]	0.38	0.36	0.0	0.03	0.14	0.21	0.29
Most people . . .			TRUST IN FELLOW MEN				
. . . can be trusted[d]	0.37	0.60	3.6	4.2	4.9	5.4	6.9
. . . try to be fair[d]	0.46	0.64	4.3	4.9	5.5	6.0	7.0
. . . try to be helpful[d]	0.42	0.56	3.6	4.2	4.9	5.6	6.2
			TRUST IN INSTITUTIONS				
Parties[b]	0.25	0.31	5.5	11.8	19.0	27.7	40.8
Justice/legal system[b]	0.35	0.64	19.9	37.7	46.4	64.6	85.8
Administration[b]	0.24	0.43	23.1	38.9	49.3	63.5	80.3
Government[b]	0.19	0.42	15.5	27.5	34.4	49.7	68.1
Parliament[b]	0.36	0.57	13.4	23.2	32.3	47.5	65.7

[a]The underlying R data frame and the complete correlation matrix are available at https://github.com/viewsandinsights/AI

$N = 21$ to 28 countries. Data sources: [b]Eurobarometer 92.3 for 2019; [c]Eurostat; [d]European Social Survey Round 9 for 2018

constitute a frequency distribution whose summary statistics (first, second, and third quartile) appear in the present Table 2.1.

The same logic applies to the covariates in Table 2.1—for instance, to the five scales that indicate the trust people have in their country's institutions. Eurobarometer 92.3 asked respondents to indicate if they tend to trust or not trust some institutions (survey question "QA6a"). Each referring to the respondent's country, the selection involved the "political parties," "justice/legal system," "public administration," "government," and the "parliament." Again using weighted frequency distributions, the respective percentage of those who tend to trust an institution (vs. tend not to trust and don't know) characterize each country, and Table 2.1 displays the summary statistics for each of the resulting five country-level variables on trust in institutions. They also reveal substantial variation across EU countries.

Trust in the institutions of one's country turns out to be a relevant covariate of the preference for public policy intervention. In principle, this applies to all five institutions but particularly to the legal system and the parliament. The higher a country's percentage of trust in these institutions, the higher is its percentage in favor of public policy intervention in said regard ($r = 0.64$ and $r = 0.57$, respectively). In essence, this result will likely mean that to ensure ethical development of AI applications, advocating state regulation requires sufficient trust in the legal system and the state. Accordingly, the population shares do correspond at the country level.

2.2.3.2 Concerns that AI Could Lead to Discrimination

Following the above Delphi scenario was a request to the respondents to rate a series of ethical aspects. From the perspective of the reference year 2030, one of these ratings addressed possible discrimination against job seekers in the labor market: "Since AI made decisions about recruiting, discrimination, stigmatization, and violation of personal rights when looking for a job have decreased significantly." We asked this because it would be very possible to use ethically acceptable programming to ensure that when looking for a job, for example, only the applicant's qualifications count. However, the respondents considered this unlikely. In contrast, they regarded the following scenario as being possible to quite probable: "Since becoming AI-driven, the classification of creditworthiness not only includes characteristics of the loan seeker himself decisions on loans have been increasingly challenged in courts in recent years."

European Countries Differ Substantially in the Percentage of Concerned People

Discrimination and creditworthiness are two topics that Eurobarometer 92.3 also addresses. The survey asked respondents if they were "concerned that the use of artificial intelligence could lead to discrimination in terms of age, gender, race, or nationality, for example in taking decisions on recruitment, creditworthiness, etc." (survey question QF3_1). We pursue the same aggregate-data measurement strategy and describe each country by its percentage of people concerned in each respect.

Concerns that the use of AI could lead to discrimination

Proportion of respondents who confirm that the use of AI could lead to discimination in terms of age, gender, race or nationality, for example in taking decisions on recruitment, creditworthiness etc

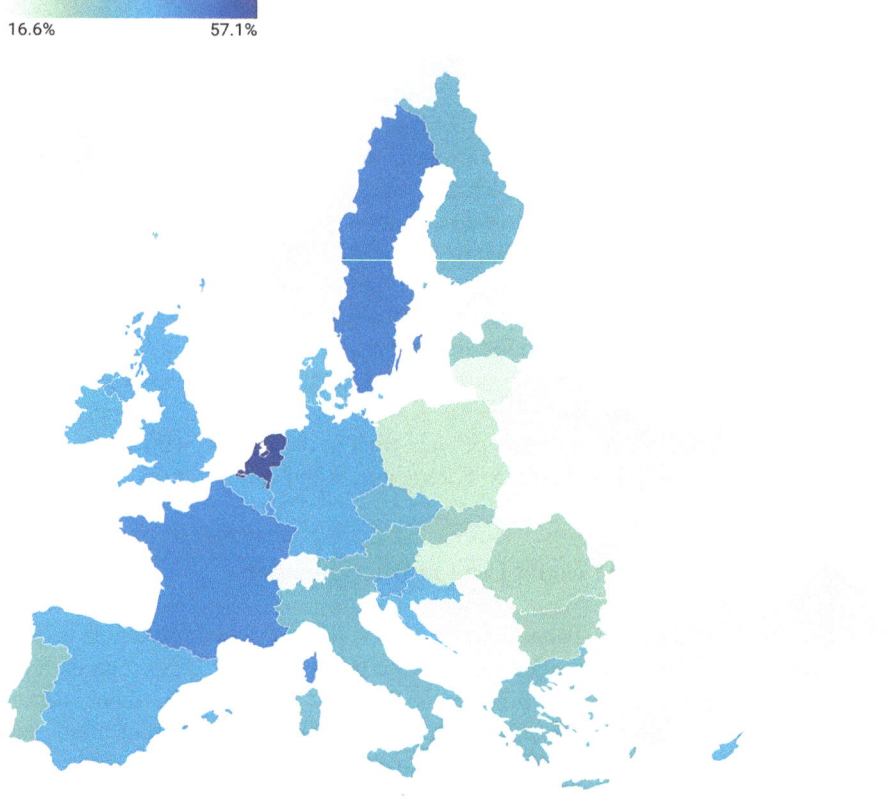

Map: Uwe Engel (University of Bremen) • Source: Eurobarometer 92.3 • Created with Datawrapper

Fig. 2.4 Concerns that the use of AI could lead to discrimination

Table 2.1 displays the summary statistics of the pertinent frequency distribution, and Table 2.3 in the appendix to this chapter reports the percentages for each involved country. We see that the smallest percentage of concerned people is 16.6 (Estonia) and the largest is 57.1 (Netherlands). We also see that the middle 50% of the values of this frequency distribution are in the range of 27.4 to 38.6, with a mean value (median) of 34.2% concerned people. Figure 2.4 graphs the EU countries in terms of this concern that the use of AI could lead to discrimination.

What explains the considerable differences among the 28 European countries? We remain at the country level and include three additional groups of aggregate variables: the country's level of prosperity and its inherent risk of poverty, the degree of multi-ethnicity, and trust in fellow men.

Covariate Measures Underlying the Correlation Analysis
Following Eurostat, we measured living standards in three ways. The first calculates living standards by measuring the price of certain goods and services in each country, relative to income in that country. Eurostat[3] explains this measure as follows: "This is done using a common national currency called the purchasing power standard (PPS). Comparing gross domestic product (GDP) per inhabitant in PPS provides an overview of living standards across the EU." We have taken over the index values Eurostat reports, showing the associated summary statistics in Table 2.1. The same goes for another measure, the poverty risk, i.e., the percentage of people at risk of poverty or social exclusion.[4] A third official measure is the material deprivation[5] rate for 2020,[6] with information from the EU-SILC survey. Eurostat explains this measure: "The indicator is defined as the percentage of population with an enforced lack of at least three out of nine material deprivation items in the 'economic strain and durables' dimension."[7]

In addition, we calculated a fourth measure using information from the European Social Survey (ESS), Round 9, for 2018. It reflects the respondent's rating of household income in terms of possible feelings of deprivation (ESS Round 9 Source Questionnaire, p. 60, survey question F42). The ESS asked which of four descriptions "comes closest to how you feel about your household's income nowadays? Living comfortably on present income (1), coping on present income (2), finding it difficult on present income (3), and finding it very difficult on present income (4)." We recoded (3) and (4) into one category and computed its percentage per country, each based on the weighted frequency distribution. For that, we used the recommended post-stratification weight.[8]

Trust in fellow men is another relevant covariate of the concern that AI could lead to discrimination. We use three 11-point rating scales from Round 9 of the European Social Survey (ESS Round 9 Source Questionnaire, p. 5, survey questions A4 to A6). We asked respondents to indicate if "most people can be trusted" (scale score: 10) or if "you can't be too careful in dealing with people" (scale score: 0). Also, respondents were asked if they think "that most people would try to take advantage of you if they got the chance" (score: 0), or if they would "try to be fair?" (score: 10). Then, respondents were to indicate if they "would say that most of the time people try to be helpful" (score: 10) or "they are mostly looking out for themselves" (score: 0). We stayed with the original scale directions toward "can be trusted," "try to be

---

[3] https://european-union.europa.eu/principles-countries-history/key-facts-and-figures/life-eu_en
[4] https://ec.europa.eu/eurostat/databrowser/view/ilc_peps01$DV_566/default/table
[5] https://ec.europa.eu/eurostat/databrowser/view/tessi080/default/table
[6] Figures for 2020 taken. Concerning Italy, figure for 2019 is substituted for the missing value for 2020.
[7] https://ec.europa.eu/eurostat/databrowser/view/tessi080/default/table
[8] The so-called pspwght weight

fair," and "try to be helpful," computing the mean value of each pertinent country-related distribution (again, using the "pspwght" survey weight).

Finally, we approached ethnicity with a survey question from Round 9 of the European Social Survey, asking respondents how they would describe their "ancestry," in terms of descent or family origins (ESS Round 9 Source Questionnaire, p. 72, survey question F61). Following recommended practice, we recoded all responses to the European Standard Classification of Cultural and Ethnic Groups available in ESS9 Appendix A6,[9] pp. 28–38, computing the pertaining "pspwght"-weighted country-related distributions and using their relative frequencies for the construction of a multi-ethnicity index. We applied two statistical formulas for this purpose, entropy and the Herfindahl index. Both formulas measure concentration. They produce their smallest index value when all cases concentrate on just one of the categories of a frequency distribution, and they attain their maximum value when the cases are evenly distributed. We compute both measures in their standardized variant as relative entropy

$$\text{RH} = \frac{-\sum_{i=1}^{I} \ln(p_i) \cdot p_i}{\ln(I)}$$

and as normalized "Herfindahl"

$$\text{RHF} = \frac{I}{I-1} \cdot \left(1 - \sum_{i=1}^{I} p_i^2\right),$$

where I indicates the number of categories, so that the resulting index values range between min $= 0$ (one-point distribution) and max $= 1$ (uniform distribution), respectively.

Correlations at the Country Level

Table 2.1 reports a consistent finding in line with Inglehart's post-materialism hypothesis of sociological value research. Higher (post-material) needs only arise when elementary (material) basic needs are satisfied. In psychological terms, the hypothesis assumes Maslow's hierarchy of needs. For instance, for someone who struggles daily for his economic existence, ethical concerns about AI-related discrimination would accordingly be an expression of such a "higher" and, thus, likely deferred need. At the aggregate level, this hypothesis should by and large imply just the observation made in the present analysis, namely, the higher a country's living standard, the higher its inherent percentage of people concerned that AI could lead to discrimination ($r = 0.5$). Correspondingly, a country's risk of poverty and deprivation correlates negatively with its share of concerned people. For example, dealing

---

[9] https://www.europeansocialsurvey.org/docs/round9/survey/ESS9_appendix_a6_e02_0.pdf

with ethical questions of AI leading to discrimination evidently tends to presuppose a life of prosperity and economic security. To exaggerate, anyone struggling for their daily economic existence probably has other concerns than possible discrimination through AI. Paradoxically, however, a possible substitution due to AI could affect just this part of the population more than others in the labor market.

In this connection, the strong positive correlation of a country's living standard with the expression of mean trust in fellow men is especially worth mentioning. As documented in the repository at github.com, referenced above, the correlations are $r = 0.65$ (trusted), 0.68 (fair), and 0.74 (helpful). Furthermore, mean trust in fellow men consistently correlates negatively and equally substantially with the deprivation measures, and slightly weaker with a country's inherent poverty risk. Stated briefly, the higher a country's deprivation and poverty-risk shares are, the smaller is its corresponding mean trust in fellow men. This is noteworthy because it indicates a relevant source of lacking or underdeveloped trust: unfavorable experiences in the daily competition for status and resources, both in economic and social regards. This becomes more understandable by attending to the opposite poles, namely, that "one can't be too careful in dealing with people," "most people would try to take advantage of others," "people are mostly looking out for themselves"—in short, a typical competitive experience. And, as Table 2.1 correlations indicate, the experience entails less concern about AI as a technology that could lead to discrimination.

Finally, structural differentiation, in terms of ethnicity (family origins), turns out to be a relevant covariate of the concern about potentially discriminatory AI applications. As Table 2.1 shows, both indices correlate positively with this concern. This means that structurally more heterogenous countries also tend to have larger shares of people with concerns about AI as a possible discriminatory instrument. This may mean that populations in structurally more heterogeneous countries are more sensitive to the issue of discrimination.

2.2.3.3 Concerns that AI Could Lead to Discrimination: the German Case

Looking inside Germany, Fig. 2.5 reveals some variation across its federal states in the concern that AI could lead to discrimination. At first glance, the spread appears considerable, ranging from 14% in Saxony-Anhalt to 67% in Bremen. However, it shows only partial statistically significant variation around the overall mean of all federal states, which the baseline odds of model 1 estimate (Table 2.2)

$$\text{Baseline odds} = \frac{Pr(\text{concerned})}{1 - Pr(\text{concerned})} = e^{b_0}$$

and the federal state in which a respondent lives multiplicatively modifies. Such a factor represents an odds ratio that further modifies the baseline, the more the factor deviates from 1.0 (= no impact).

Concerns that the use of AI could lead to discrimination

Proportion of respondents who confirm they have concerns that the use of AI could lead to discrimination in terms of age, gender, race or nationality, for example in taking decisions on recruitment, creditworthiness etc.

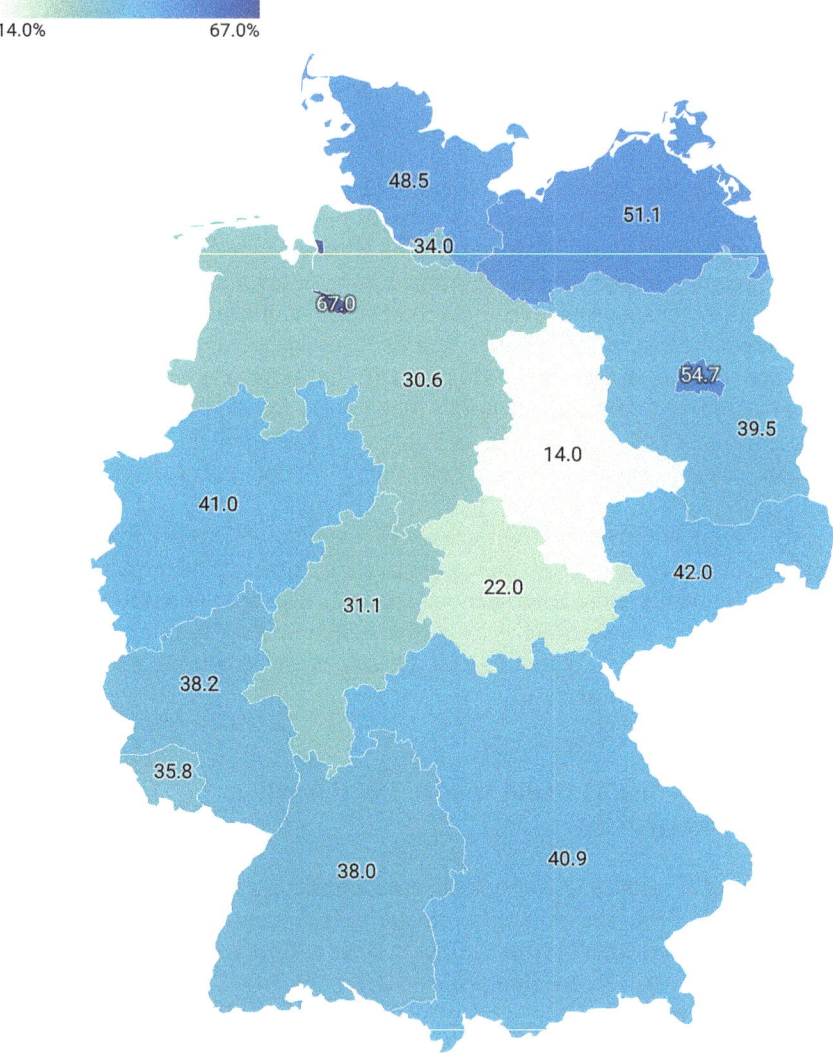

Map: Uwe Engel (University of Bremen) • Source: Eurobarometer 92.3 • Created with Datawrapper

Fig. 2.5 Concerns that AI could lead to discrimination, by Federal states of Germany

$$\frac{Pr(\text{concerned}|\text{federal state})}{1 - Pr(\text{concerned}|\text{federal state})} = e^{b_0} \times e^{b_{\text{federal state}}}.$$

Table 2.2 reports these odds ratios along with the pertinent significance information. Using the usual two-tailed $b/s.e \geq |1.96|$ criterion, only four federal states deviate significantly from the baseline odds, e^{b_0}, namely, Bremen, Berlin, Thuringia, and Saxony-Anhalt.

We deal with the social structure of said "concern" in the enlarged logistic regression equation of model 2. It replenishes the set of explanatory variables with information about gender, age, social class, and education. In this equation, too, the federal states show statistically significant spread around the overall mean for a subset of such states. Net of the effect of gender, age, social class, and education, significant spread remains for Bremen, Berlin, and Saxony-Anhalt. While Thuringia loses statistical significance in this enlarged equation, now Mecklenburg–Western Pomerania and Lower Saxony join the list. While such significant variation involves federal states of the former East and West Germany equally well, we observe a clear East/West difference in terms of the preference for public policy intervention to ensure that AI develops in an ethical manner. In this regard, the percentages are 65% for the West and 52% for East Germany.

According to model 2, some factors, in addition to federal state, that modify the baseline odds multiplicatively significantly modify the odds of having concerns that AI could lead to discrimination. This set of factors includes gender (women), age in years, and social class, whereas the respondent's age when he/she stopped full-time education (higher education, as measured by age education 20+ vs. rest) contributes only insignificantly to the equation.

$$\text{Odds}(\text{concerned}) = e^{b_0} \times e^{b_{\text{federal state}}}$$
$$\times e^{b_{\text{gender}}} \times e^{b_{\text{age} \times \text{years}}} \times e^{b_{\text{age}^2 \times \text{years}^2}} \times e^{b_{\text{social class}}} \times e^{b_{\text{education}}}.$$

Using 1.0 as a benchmark indicating "no impact," the factors (odds ratios) in Table 2.2 show, for instance, how these factors modify the odds of having concerns. Examples appear among women who are at 0.68 times the odds among men and 1.5 times larger among the middle (vs. working) class. In this connection, "concern" and age relate nonlinearly. This proves the coefficients for age and age-squared, evident by plotting the percentage of concern against six age groups, each covering a 10-year span. Then, the percentage runs from 29.8 in the youngest age group 15+; over 37.0, and 37.8 up to 48.6 in the group aged 45+; falling again to over 40.9 and 35.3 in the group aged 65 + .

2.3 Trust in the State and Ethical Concerns of the Secured and Wealthy

The competitive scenario of a destructive human–robot competition for permanent appointments would hit the well-educated middle class particularly hard. Following the *expert opinions*, such cutthroat competition appears as an unlikely worst-case scenario. But what if, contrary to expectations, it did happen in the future? Then, the Delphi respondents consider four sociological implications likely: increased importance of education as the key to professional success, demand for lifelong tax-financed protection of an acceptable livelihood, political weakening of the liberal center in favor of the fringes of the spectrum, and increased demand for psychosocial counseling.

But how does the *population* see it? In short, only a minority considers itself replaceable in the job, and relatively more people expect positive, not negative AI-related effects on their standard of living and quality of life. All in all, the personal concern appears limited.

AI trustworthiness is a big issue, including its ethically acceptable programming. Therefore, finding out how much AI encounters ethical concerns in the population is of vital interest. Based on data from EU statistics and European social research, an aggregate data analysis at the country level shows that ethical concerns do exist; the more prosperous a country or the more economically secure its population, the more that is true. The analysis suggests (for example) that dealing with ethical questions so that AI could lead to discrimination tends to presuppose a life of prosperity and economic security. It also suggests a negative correlation between the personal experience of having to sustain one's position in the daily competition for status and resources and concerns about AI as a technology that could lead to discrimination. The struggle for daily economic existence will trigger concerns other than possible discrimination through AI.

A survey data analysis for Germany reveals a social-class effect on the odds of ethical concerns that also indicates the relevance of post-materialism. The analysis shows particularly that belonging to the middle class increases these odds. Compared to the working class, the odds ratios are all significantly greater than 1.0 for the lower-middle, middle, upper-middle, and higher classes. In addition, the curvilinear age effect may indirectly indicate a sensitivity to discrimination, reflecting typical biographical experiences in occupational life courses.

The analysis shows a preference for regulation. The European population was asked about the need for public policy intervention, the ability of industry providers of Artificial Intelligence to deal with these issues themselves, or if ensuring that Artificial Intelligence applications are developed ethically requires no specific action. The figures reveal a clearly propagated need for regulation to be met by either state or industry, with a clear preference for state regulation. However, with substantial differences between the EU countries, a significant covariate, namely, trust in the institutions of one's country, turns out to be a relevant covariate of the preference for public policy intervention, particularly trust in the legal system and the parliament.

Table 2.2 Concern that AI could lead to discrimination: structural factors of impact

	Concern %	Logistic regression equations			
		Model 1		Model 2	
		Odds ratio	b/se	Odds ratio	b/se
Baseline odds		0.63	−5.86	0.11	−5.38
Federal state and socio-demography					
Bremen	67	3.25	2.09	3.1	1.98
Berlin	54.7	1.93	2.7	1.88	2.54
Mecklenburg–Western Pomerania	51.1	1.67	1.47	2.14	2.09
Schleswig-Holstein	48.5	1.5	1.54	1.47	1.41
Saxony	42	1.16	0.64	1.26	0.97
North Rhine-Westphalia	41	1.11	0.8	1.08	0.54
Bavaria	40.9	1.11	0.7	1.15	0.94
Brandenburg	39.5	1.04	0.15	1	−0.01
Rhineland-Palatinate	38.2	0.99	−0.04	0.86	−0.61
Baden-Wuerttemberg	38	0.98	−0.11	0.95	−0.29
Saarland	35.8	0.89	−0.25	0.82	−0.44
Hamburg	34	0.83	−0.55	0.8	−0.64
Hesse	31.1	0.72	−1.6	0.74	−1.42
Lower Saxony	30.6	0.7	−1.89	0.63	−2.44
Thuringia	22	0.45	−2.19	0.52	−1.73
Saxony-Anhalt	14	0.26	−3.18	0.27	−3.06
Gender (Women)				0.68	−3.59
Age				1.069	4.09
Age(squared)				0.999	−4.02
Lower-middle class				1.92	3.26
Middle class				1.5	2.33
Upper-middle and higher class				1.88	2.6
Other				0.9	−0.24
Age education 20+				1.19	1.42

$N = 1540$. Eurobarometer survey weight for Germany ("w3") used. The table displays, for each federal state of Germany, the percentage of concerned persons as also shown in Fig. 2.5. In addition, the table reports the estimated odds ratios for two logistic regression models. Effect coding is used for the federal states to obtain their estimates as deviations around their overall mean. The *complete* set of estimates, i.e., including those for the reference category, is obtained by estimating each model twice, for instance, once with Lower Saxony and once with North Rhine-Westphalia taken as reference category. This is a straightforward way of obtaining a standard-error estimate of the reference category's b, while this b itself is simply the negative sum of all other b's in the equation. Dummy coding is used for gender (reference category: men), social class (reference category: working class), and education (reference category: all other categories except for the explicit "20+" category). A polynomial regression is involved in terms of age and age-squared. Data source: Eurobarometer 92.3.

Appendix

Table 2.3 Preference for public policy intervention and concern that AI could lead to discrimination, by European countries

		Row percent (QF4)				Percent
		Public policy	Industry providers	No action needed	Other	Concern (Qf3_1)
NL	Netherlands	77.5	6.5	4.3	11.7	57.1
SE	Sweden	71.7	8.7	3.4	16.3	46.5
DE-W	Germany (West)	65.0	11.1	4.5	19.4	38.5
DK	Denmark	62.9	7.4	5.9	23.8	36.2
DE*	Germany (all)	62.4	11.7	4.7	21.2	38.5
FI	Finland	59.8	14.0	5.4	20.9	33.8
LU	Luxembourg	57.8	8.7	5.3	28.2	42.2
GB	United Kingdom	57.1	11.6	4.9	26.4	39.4
FR	France	56.5	10.0	5.3	28.2	44.6
CY	Cyprus	56.1	10.8	7.3	25.8	37
DE-E	Germany (East)	51.6	14.1	5.8	28.5	38.8
GR	Greece	51.3	23.7	5.0	20.0	31.9
IT	Italy	51.0	18.0	8.5	22.5	32.7
IE	Ireland	50.0	24.3	5.2	20.6	37.9
ES	Spain	49.8	12.7	4.5	33.0	38.4
BE	Belgium	49.3	21.5	10.1	19.0	38.8
SI	Slovenia	47.7	12.9	8.6	30.8	38.9
EU	*Overall*	*46.6*	*18.1*	*8.4*	*27.0*	*33.5*
PT	Portugal	45.6	19.1	7.1	28.3	29.3
LT	Lithuania	40.0	18.6	7.2	34.2	19.4
EE	Estonia	39.8	14.5	7.3	38.4	16.6
AT	Austria	39.6	22.4	13.0	25.0	32
BG	Bulgaria	33.8	18.7	5.0	42.5	26.4
MT	Malta	33.7	12.8	8.7	44.9	23.4
CZ	Czech Republic	33.4	20.7	12.9	33.1	34.5
LV	Latvia	33.4	17.0	16.5	33.2	28.5
HR	Croatia	32.6	26.7	11.2	29.5	37
SK	Slovakia	31.4	27.0	11.5	30.2	27.7
PL	Poland	31.3	25.1	15.7	27.9	22.3
HU	Hungary	29.7	33.0	12.5	24.7	21.1
RO	Romania	19.0	38.5	16.4	26.1	25.6

W1-weighted frequency distribution, except for the w3-weighted distributions for DE* Germany (all). Data source: Eurobarometer 92.3 for Nov./Dec. of 2019. Country-specific percentage bases for almost all countries around 1000, except for Germany (all, with $N = 1540$) and Luxembourg, Cyprus, Germany (East), and Malta (with around 500 cases each). Overall N for EU is 27,382.

(continued)

Question wording (QF4): "Which statement below do you agree most to finish the statement: To ensure that Artificial Intelligence applications are developed in an ethical manner . . . public policy intervention is needed [1], . . . industry providers of Artificial Intelligence can deal with these issues themselves [2], . . . no specific action is needed [3], Other (SPONTANEOUS) [4], None of the above [5], Don't know [6]." [ ] added. In the table above categories 4, 5, and 6 are recoded to "Other" and included in the percentage bases. In Fig. 2.3, categories 4, 5, and 6 have been excluded from computing the relative frequencies (proportions). Question wording (QF3_1): "Which statements below, if any, would you select to finish the statement: You are concerned that the use of artificial intelligence could lead to . . . discrimination in terms of age, gender, race, or nationality, for example in taking decisions on recruitment, creditworthiness, etc." The table above indicates the percentages of respondents "concerned" in this regard. Please note that the summary statistics and correlations reported above in Table 2.1 consider only the values for Germany (all) and not the values shown for Germany East and West

References

Adams-Prassl, J. (2019). What if your boss was an algorithm? Economic incentives, legal challenges, and the rise of artificial intelligence at work. *Comparative Labor Law and Policy Journal, 41*, 123. Retrieved December 29, 2021, from https://papers.ssrn.com/sol3/papers.cfm?abstract_id=3661151

Aghion, P., Jones, B. F., & Jones, C. I. (2019). 9. *Artificial intelligence and economic growth* (pp. 237–290). University of Chicago Press.

Baldwin, R. (2019). *The globotics upheaval. Globalisation, robotics, and the future of work*. Weidenfeld & Nicolson.

Bankins, S., & Formosa, P. (2020). When AI meets PC: Exploring the implications of workplace social robots and a human-robot psychological contract. *European Journal of Work and Organizational Psychology, 29*(2), 215–229.

Decker, M., Fischer, M., & Ott, I. (2017). Service robotics and human labor: A first technology assessment of substitution and cooperation. *Robotics and Autonomous Systems, 87*, 348–354.

Engel, U., & Dahlhaus, L. (2022). Data quality and privacy concerns in digital trace data. In U. Engel, A. Quan-Haase, S. Liu, & L. Lyberg (Eds.), *Handbook of computational social science, Vol. 1 - Theory, case studies and ethics* (pp. 343–362). Routledge. https://doi.org/10.4324/9781003024583-23

European Commission. (2019, November–December). *Brussels: Eurobarometer 92.3, 2019. Kantar Public, Brussels [Producer]*. GESIS, Cologne [Publisher]: ZA7601, dataset version 1.0.0. Retrieved from https://doi.org/10.4232/1.13564

European Commission & European Parliament. (2017, March). *Brussels: Eurobarometer 87.1, March 2017. TNS opinion, Brussels [Producer]*. GESIS, Cologne [Publisher]: ZA6861, data set version 1.2.0. Retrieved from https://doi.org/10.4232/1.12922

European Social Survey. (2018). *ESS round 9 source questionnaire*. Retrieved from ERIC Headquarters c/o City, University of London. Retrieved from https://www.europeansocialsurvey.org/

Felten, E., Raj, M., & Seamans, R. (2018). A method to link advances in artificial intelligence to occupational abilities. *AEA Papers and Proceedings, 108*, 54–57.

Ferrer, X., van Nuenen, T., Such, J. M., Coté, M., & Criado, N. (2021). Bias and discrimination in AI: A cross-disciplinary perspective. *IEEE Technology and Society Magazine, 40*(2), 72–80.

Ford, M. (2016). *The rise of the robots. Technology and the threat of mass unemployment*. Oneworld Publications.

Frank, M. R., Autor, D., Bessen, J. E., Brynjolfsson, E., Cebrian, M., Deming, D. J., Feldman, M., Groh, M., Lobo, J., Moro, E., Wang, D., & Youn, H.& Rahwan, I. (2019). Toward understanding the impact of artificial intelligence on labor. *Proceedings of the National Academy of Sciences, 116*(14), 6531–6539.

Goffart, D. (2019). Das Ende der Mittelschicht, wie wir sie kennen. *Focus 12/19, 16*, 52–59.

Graetz, G., & Michaels, G. (2015). *Robots at work, CEP Discussion Papers, Centre for Economic Performance, LSE*. Retrieved December 30, 2021, from https://EconPapers.repec.org/RePEc:cep:cepdps:dp1335

Hamid, O. H., Smith, N. L., & Barzanji, A. (2017, July). Automation, per se, is not job elimination: How artificial intelligence forwards cooperative human-machine coexistence. In *2017 IEEE 15th International Conference on Industrial Informatics (INDIN)* (pp. 899–904). IEEE.

Huang, M. H., & Rust, R. T. (2018). Artificial intelligence in service. *Journal of Service Research, 21*(2), 155–172.

Keynes, J. M. (2010 [1930]). Economic possibilities for our grandchildren. In *Essays in persuasion* (pp. 321–332). Palgrave Macmillan.

Kleinberg, J., Ludwig, J., Mullainathan, S., & Sunstein, C. R. (2020). Algorithms as discrimination detectors. *Proceedings of the National Academy of Sciences, 117*(48), 30096–30100.

Lane, M., & Saint-Martin, A. (2021). The impact of Artificial Intelligence on the labour market: What do we know so far? In *OECD Social, Employment and Migration Working Papers, No. 256*. OECD. https://doi.org/10.1787/7c895724-en

Operto, S. (2019). Evaluating public opinion towards robots: A mixed-method approach. *Paladyn, Journal of Behavioral Robotics, 10*, 286–297. https://doi.org/10.1515/pjbr-2019-0023

Webb, M. (2019). The impact of artificial intelligence on the labor market. *Economics of Innovation eJournal*. https://doi.org/10.2139/ssrn.3482150

Wrobel, M., & Althoff, J. (2021). *Entwicklung der Substituierbarkeitspotenziale auf dem Arbeitsmarkt in Niedersachsen und Bremen von 2013 bis 2019*. IAB-Regional 1|2021. Institut für Arbeitsmarkt- und Berufsforschung (Institute for Employment Research, Nuremberg, Germany]. Retrieved from https://doku.iab.de/regional/NSB/2021/regional_nsb_0121.pdf

Uwe Engel is a Professor at the University of Bremen (Germany), where he held a chair in sociology from 2000 until his retirement in autumn 2020. In 2007, he founded the Social Science Methods Centre of Bremen University, and directed this institution until 2020. Current work focuses on computational social science and human–robot interaction. See https://www.viewsandinsights.com/en/welcome-to-views-insights and https://orcid.org/0000-0001-8420-9677 for details.

Lena Dahlhaus is a lecturer at the Carl von Ossietzky University of Oldenburg, where she teaches social science methods and statistical data analysis. Following a bachelor's degree in Sociology, she received a master's degree in Social Research with distinction from the University of Bremen in 2020. Previously, Lena has been working at the Social Science Methods Centre and the Working Group Statistics and Social Research at the University of Bremen, where she was involved in research projects about the role of Artificial Intelligence in society. Her research interests include Survey Methodology, Natural Language Processing, research ethics, and the integration of traditional and new forms of data.

Open Access This chapter is licensed under the terms of the Creative Commons Attribution 4.0 International License (http://creativecommons.org/licenses/by/4.0/), which permits use, sharing, adaptation, distribution and reproduction in any medium or format, as long as you give appropriate credit to the original author(s) and the source, provide a link to the Creative Commons license and indicate if changes were made.

The images or other third party material in this chapter are included in the chapter's Creative Commons license, unless indicated otherwise in a credit line to the material. If material is not included in the chapter's Creative Commons license and your intended use is not permitted by statutory regulation or exceeds the permitted use, you will need to obtain permission directly from the copyright holder.

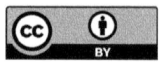

Chapter 3
The Bremen AI Delphi Study

Uwe Engel and Lena Dahlhaus

Abstract The chapter introduces the Bremen AI Delphi study, recently conducted in Germany's city-state of Bremen. This study consists of a large Delphi survey of scientists from different backgrounds and involves a subsample of stakeholders from politics ($N = 297$ participants). The study consists also of a closely related population survey ($N = 216$ participants). The chapter describes sampling and survey design and introduces basic features of questionnaire architecture.

Keywords Real-time Delphi survey · Bremen AI Delphi Study · Online survey · Test-retest design · Opinion formation · Sample and survey design · Questionnaire design · Standard response scale

3.1 Introduction

If researching current trends already involves real challenges, predicting future trends holds even more. Predictions are usually difficult to make and inherently uncertain. However, the Delphi method makes it possible to quantify this uncertainty by gathering many expert opinions on a future issue. We can then easily see how much these assessments differ from one another or resemble each other. The method also provides the possibility of reducing the uncertainty, at least in principle, by asking the experts in a Delphi for their assessments not just once but repeatedly. The process confronts them with the statistical results from the previous survey round and asks them to reassess their previous responses in light of these results. The experts can then either stick to their earlier assessment or change it, and we can see whether and how much the expert opinions converge across survey rounds. Thus, the

---

U. Engel (✉)
University of Bremen, Bremen, Germany
e-mail: uengel@uni-bremen.de

L. Dahlhaus
University of Oldenburg, Oldenburg, Germany
e-mail: lena.dahlhaus@uol.de

© The Author(s) 2023
U. Engel (ed.), *Robots in Care and Everyday Life*, SpringerBriefs in Sociology,
https://doi.org/10.1007/978-3-031-11447-2_3

feedback between rounds facilitates informed decision-making in the process (Linstone & Turoff, 2011). In a conventional Delphi, this process can occur across several survey rounds; in a real-time Online-Delphi, one such round is sufficient to obtain an assessment along with one reassessment, the approach the present study pursues.

A Delphi has no group discussion in a socio-psychological sense. All experts remain anonymous during the entire Delphi process, and not interacting rules out any group dynamics that could affect the expert opinions—a great advantage. However, this same design feature also precludes achieving through discussion a shared understanding of the target in question. Thus, designing and wording the survey questions to ensure comparability of answers in even the most complex subject matter is of utmost importance. The present study accomplishes this by establishing a sequence for each of five complex scenarios (Engel & Schultheis 2021). First, we ask respondents for a response to a complex scenario that consists of multiple dimensions; then, we use follow-up scales to assess each such dimension separately. While the complex scenario helps to convey to the respondent a realistic idea of the imagined future situation and a basis for empathizing with it, the follow-up scales help to ensure precise and comparable responses.

The appropriate selection of experts is an extremely important task for a Delphi. It must ensure the competent assessment of all relevant aspects of the subject matter in question. We describe this selection for the present study in the next section. Its basis is the preference for a larger rather than a smaller selection of experts, as well for a sufficiently heterogeneous group of experts able to cover the topic of "AI and society" from the point of view of various relevant groups. Finally, belonging to the Free Hanseatic City of Bremen as the scientific location is a eligibility criterion for all the participating scientists.

In the past, Delphi surveys have been the method of choice to forecast future societal changes in a variety of research agendas. For several decades in Germany, Delphi surveys have provided decision-makers with valuable insights into ongoing and future trends. For example, the German Federal Ministry of Education and Research (BMBF) first conducted Delphi studies[1] in 1992, 1993, and 1998, to assess societal trends and challenges for science and technology. Their results culminated in policy recommendations, participative studies, and the still ongoing "Foresight" cycles that focus on development trends with a view toward the year 2030.

The "Foresight" study, a large-scale multinational Delphi survey and part of the BOHEMIA study,—recently carried out for the European Commission, in preparation of the next research framework program, 2021–2027 Horizon Europe (European Commission, 2018)—offered only a first rough orientation for the development of scenarios for the present study. A detailed study of human–robot interaction required developing a completely new, precise, and detailed instrument for the present Bremen AI Delphi study.

---

[1] https://www.bmbf.de/bmbf/de/forschung/zukunftstrends/foresight/foresight-als-methode-der-strategischen-vorausschau-im-bmbf/foresight-als-methode-der-strategischen-vorausschau-im-bmbf_node.html

3.2 Sample and Survey Design

3.2.1 Delphi Survey of Scientists and Stakeholders

As outlined elsewhere (Engel & Dahlhaus, 2022), we invited 1826 experts from two different backgrounds to participate in the Bremen AI Delphi Study, namely 1359 members of Bremen's scientific community and a diverse group of 467 people on Bremen's political landscape. The expert group from the Bremen scientific community included scientists affiliated with one of Bremen's public or private universities at the time of the survey. The prerequisite for participation was holding a doctorate or a professorship.

Disciplines from the social sciences included economics, sociology, political science, health science/public health, cultural science, pedagogy, media and communication science, linguistics, psychology, philosophy, and history. Professionals in engineering, mathematics, robotics, and computer science represented the STEM disciplines. The natural sciences included physics, chemistry, biology, and earth science. The group of political experts, including officials and stakeholders, comprised members of the Bremen Parliament (all party affiliations) and officials serving in senate departments. The group of stakeholders included union representatives, executives of organizations of employer representation, and pastors of Bremen's Catholic and Protestant parishes. The Delphi sample achieved a response rate of 17.8% ($n = 297$).

3.2.2 Population Survey

Following a quasi-randomization approach (Elliott & Valliant, 2017), the overall sample consisted of a combined probability and nonprobability sample. A probability sample of residents aged 18+ was drawn from the population register of the municipality of Bremen, weighted for unit-nonresponse, and used as a reference sample for the estimation of inclusion probabilities for an analog volunteer sample. The response rate of the probability sample was 2.5%. Sample sizes were 108 cases each, so the overall N was 216 people, aged 18 and over. Throughout this book, all analyses of the population survey are based on weighted frequency distributions to balance nonresponse. The weighting approach devised for this is detailed in a recent freely accessible handbook chapter (Engel & Dahlhaus, 2022, pp. 356–357).

3.2.3 Fieldwork

Fieldwork for the two surveys took place from 25 November to 15 December 2019. Invitations to the Delphi were sent via personalized e-mail to the recipient's professional address, and if no response was received within 2 weeks, reminders were sent. Invitation to the population survey was conveyed via personalized letter post, including a link to the web questionnaire (probability sample), an advertisement in the local newspapers, and an announcement on the homepage of the University of Bremen website (volunteer sample).

3.3 Questionnaire Design

3.3.1 The Scenarios for the Reference Year of 2030

A Delphi functions on the processing of the answers to survey questions to present the statistical findings to the respondents again in the succeeding round. In a conventional Delphi, this procedure takes place in separate survey rounds; in a real-time Delphi, within one such round. This reduces the otherwise likely three-to-five survey rounds to a test–retest design, thus limiting the capability of mapping the process of opinion formation and assessing it for possible convergence. However, it offers the great advantage of providing the respondents with quick feedback.

Test–Retest Agreement
In the present study, we implemented the survey of scientists and stakeholders as a real-time Delphi. The related survey questions specifically concern the five Delphi scenarios embodying the themes at the intersection of AI and society: competition, wealth, communication, conflict, and assistance. For each of these scenarios, the model for phrasing questions was: "What do you expect: Will this scenario become a reality?" Then, the standard response scale used consistently throughout the surveys was: "not at all," "probably not," "possibly," "quite probable," and "quite certain." Participants first responded to the question, then received access to a text field to optionally explain their response. Next in the sequence was the presentation of the frequency distribution of all assessments to that point in the Delphi sample, followed again by the standard response scale for a renewed rating. We observed an average agreement of $\kappa = 0.8$ across the five scenarios. The definition of the weighted kappa

$$\kappa = \frac{p_o - p_e}{1 - p_e}$$

is the probability of observed matches (p_o) minus the probability of matches expected by chance (p_e), divided by one minus the probability of expected matches. Thus, κ expresses the excess of observed over expected agreement as a share of the maximal possible excess. Accordingly, a weighted κ of 0.8 indicates that the observed agreement of assessment and reassessment exceeds the expected agreement by 80% of the maximum possible excess.

3 The Bremen AI Delphi Study

Table 3.1 Expected influence of AI on one's perceived quality of life

Expected influence of AI on one's own quality of life—asked in the interview once immediately before ("pre") and once immediately after ("post") the questions about human–robot communication (total percentages of $N = 215$)

"pre" \ "post"	Positive	No	Negative	Don't know	Sum
Positive	35.81	3.72	0.93	5.12	45.58
No	6.05	17.21	2.33	0.00	25.59
Negative	0.47	0.93	10.23	0.93	12.56
Don't know	2.79	2.33	3.26	7.91	16.29
Sum	45.12	24.19	16.75	13.96	100

Cohen's weighted kappa $= 0.57$ of assessment ("pre") and reassessment ("post")

The Larger Fictitious Context and Its Single Situational Dimensions
Each scenario refers to the reference year of 2030 and follows a clear structure. In an initial block, the scenario is deliberately pictured as a larger context and not as a narrowly defined situation. This construction should make it easier for the respondents to empathize with this fictional future situation before answering. However, this desired multidimensionality of the picture requires specific follow-up questions about the single dimensions inherent in the broader picture. In a subsequent block, each respondent is asked to rate these dimensions, employing the standard response scale. Chapter 2 demonstrates this using the competitive scenario as an example.

3.3.2 Assessing the Future Without Primary Experience

The future-oriented nature of the survey questions precludes the respondents from already having relevant application experience with the technology. The ideas about robots and AI on which the answers may be based are, therefore, highly relevant. Quite conceivably, the cognitive processing of the interview questions itself helps to develop such ideas. Therefore, we asked a survey question on the expected influence of AI on one's quality of life, once immediately before and once immediately after a block of questions about communication between humans and robots, to see whether and how the answers changed under the impression from this block of questions.

Table 3.1 shows such a response effect. Even if the pre-/post-distributions differ only slightly and, thus, indicate a high level of aggregate stability, this stability goes hand-in-hand with a substantial change in individual responses. Only 71.2% of the respondents stayed with their original answers (sum of the percentages on the main diagonal). In contrast, 13% corrected an initially positive expectation toward "no influence," "negative influence," or "don't know" (sum of percentages in the upper triangle) while, at the same time, 15.8% changed their assessment in the opposite direction (lower subdiagonal triangle). The weighted κ of 0.57 indicates that the observed agreement of assessment and reassessment exceeds the expected agreement by only 57% of the maximum possible excess.

3.3.3 Randomized Sequence of Items

The presentation of unordered sets of categories should consider the "primacy" vs. "recency" distinction that Krosnick and Alwin (Weisberg, 2005, p. 108f.) identify. Accordingly, the impact of response order presumes depending on the mode of presenting the question: "With visual presentation, primacy effects will predominate; with auditory presentation, recency effects" (Tourangeau et al., 2000, p. 252). "Primacy effects" means that respondents tend to prefer options at the beginning of the list over those at the end; "recency effects" means the opposite tendency, to prefer options at the end of the list over those at the beginning (Engel, 2020, p. 248). A solution to such effects of the response order is the presentation of the list to each respondent in randomized order. This is the solution also implemented throughout the present study whenever lists of unordered items were presented to respondents.

3.3.4 The Standard Response Scale

A scale consistently employed throughout the two involved surveys, the Delphi and the population survey, ensured comparable responses. Following recommended practice from survey methodology (Schnell, 2012, p. 91f.), this standard scale rates the degree of belief in the validity of statements by using an ordinal scale. This scale maps numbers to their meanings accordingly:

1 = "not at all"
2 = "probably not"
3 = "possibly"
4 = "quite probable"
5 = "quite certain"

Using these numbers, we computed interpolated quartiles for such frequency distributions. Throughout the book, this is the respective first (Q_1), second (Q_2), and third (Q_3) quartile, to thus obtain a suitable mean estimate (Q_2 = median) and the corners of the interquartile range for the middle 50% of responses. In the chapters of this volume, we often use a standard instrument, the box plot, to graph this kind of information. In addition, the ordinal scale level is considered by specifying probit regression equations. This concerns essentially the confirmatory factor analyses in the chapters of this volume.

Figure 3.1 illustrates the interpolation scheme in the case of quartile computations. The calculation is based on two auxiliary assumptions: (1) that a scale point represents the midpoint of a surrounding interval and (2) that the responses are evenly distributed within each such interval. Then, it makes sense to determine the very share *of the class width* to be added to the relevant lower interval bound, to reach a sought quartile.

Response	1	2	3	4	5
p %	9.3	47.6	28.4	13.3	1.3
Lower bounds	0.5	1.5	2.5	3.5	4.5	5.5

class width = 1

cp %	9.3	56.9	85.3	98.6	99.9
	$cp_{i-1} \rightarrow$	$q_i - cp_{i-1}$			
		p_i			

$$Q_{i(interplated)} = lower\ bound_i + \left(\frac{Q_i - cp_{i-1}}{p_i}\right) \times class\ width$$

Q_i = 25.0 for 1st quartile, 50.0 for 2nd quartile (=median), and 75.0 for 3rd quartile

Fig. 3.1 Interpolation scheme using as example the percentages for the "competitive scenario" detailed in Chap. 2

In the present case, this class width is equal to 1. Using the percentages for the competitive scenario as an example, 9.3% have an observed score of 1 and 56.9% have an observed score of 2 or less than 2.

$$Q_{2(interplated)} = 1.5 + \left(\frac{50.0 - 9.3}{47.6}\right) \times 1 = 1.5 + 0.86 \times 1 = 2.4.$$

This implies, for instance, that the median (second quartile) falls in the interval of 1.5 to 2.5 (because this interval contains the cumulative 50% corresponding to the median), but the interval contains more than the required 50% of respondents—in fact, 56.9%. Interpolation then simply means the calculation of the portion of the class width, up to the theoretical value of 50%. In the present case, this portion is 0.86 (i.e., 86% of the whole class width of 1 is to be added to the lower interval bound).

References

Elliott, M. R., & Valliant, R. (2017). Inference for nonprobability samples. *Statistical Science, 2017*, 249–264.

Engel, U. (2020). Interest in science: Response order effects in an adaptive survey design. In A. Mays, A. Dingelstedt, V. Hambauer, S. Schlosser, F. Berens, J. Leibold, & J. Höhne (Eds.), *Grundlagen – Methoden – Anwendungen in den Sozialwissenschaften [Basics - Methods - Applications in the social sciences]* (pp. 247–261). Springer VS.

Engel, U., & Dahlhaus, L. (2022). Data quality and privacy concerns in digital trace data. In U. Engel, A. Quan-Haase, S. Liu, & L. Lyberg (Eds.), *Handbook of computational social science, Vol. 1 - Theory, case studies and ethics* (pp. 343–362). Routledge. https://doi.org/10.4324/9781003024583-23

Engel, U., & Schultheis, H. (2021). KI assistiert, der Mensch entscheidet. In A. Strasser, W. Sohst, R. Stapelfeldt, & K. Stepec (Eds.), *Künstliche Intelligenz. Die große Verheißung* (pp. 419–443). xenomoi Verlag.

European Commission. (2018). *Transitions on the Horizon: Perspectives for the European Union's future research and innovation policies*. Retrieved December 31, 2021, from https://ec.europa.eu/info/publications/transitions-horizon-perspectives-european-unions-future-research-and-innovation-policies_en

Linstone, H. A., & Turoff, M. (2011). Delphi: A brief look backward and forward. *Technological Forecasting and Social Change, 78*(9), 1712–1719.

Schnell, R. (2012). *Survey-Interviews. Methoden standardisierter Befragungen [Suvey interviews. Methods of standardized surveys]*. VS Verlag für Sozialwissenschaften/Springer Fachmedien.

Tourangeau, R., Rips, L. J., & Rasinski, K. (2000). *The psychology of survey response*. University Press.

Weisberg, H. F. (2005). *The total survey error approach. A guide to the new science of survey research*. University of Chicago Press.

Uwe Engel is a Professor at the University of Bremen (Germany), where he held a chair in sociology from 2000 until his retirement in autumn 2020. In 2007, he founded the Social Science Methods Centre of Bremen University, and directed this institution until 2020. Current work focuses on computational social science and human–robot interaction. See https://www.viewsandinsights.com/en/welcome-to-views-insights and https://orcid.org/0000-0001-8420-9677 for details.

Lena Dahlhaus is a lecturer at the Carl von Ossietzky University of Oldenburg, where she teaches social science methods and statistical data analysis. Following a bachelor's degree in Sociology, she received a master's degree in Social Research with distinction from the University of Bremen in 2020. Previously, Lena has been working at the Social Science Methods Centre and the Working Group Statistics and Social Research at the University of Bremen, where she was involved in research projects about the role of Artificial Intelligence in society. Her research interests include Survey Methodology, Natural Language Processing, research ethics, and the integration of traditional and new forms of data.

Open Access This chapter is licensed under the terms of the Creative Commons Attribution 4.0 International License (http://creativecommons.org/licenses/by/4.0/), which permits use, sharing, adaptation, distribution and reproduction in any medium or format, as long as you give appropriate credit to the original author(s) and the source, provide a link to the Creative Commons license and indicate if changes were made.

The images or other third party material in this chapter are included in the chapter's Creative Commons license, unless indicated otherwise in a credit line to the material. If material is not included in the chapter's Creative Commons license and your intended use is not permitted by statutory regulation or exceeds the permitted use, you will need to obtain permission directly from the copyright holder.

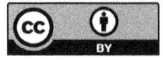

Chapter 4
The Challenge of Autonomy: What We Can Learn from Research on Robots Designed for Harsh Environments

Sirko Straube, Nina Hoyer, Niels Will, and Frank Kirchner

Abstract In addition to areas of application in people's everyday lives and the area of education and services, robots are primarily envisioned in non-immediate living environments by the society—i.e., in inaccessible or even hostile environments to humans. The results of this population survey clearly demonstrate that such application options come across with a high level of acceptance and application potential among the population. Nevertheless, it is expected that the underlying AI in such systems works reliably and that safety for humans is guaranteed.

In this chapter, the results of the study are compared with state-of-the-art systems from classical application environments for robots, like the deep-sea and space. Here, systems have to interact with their environment to a large extent on their own over longer periods of time. Although typically the designs are such that humans are able to intervene in specific situations and so external decisions are possible, the requirements for autonomy are also extremely high. From this perspective one can easily derive what kind of requirements are also necessary, and what challenges are still in front of us, when robots should be acting largely autonomous in our everyday life.

Keywords Robotics · Artificial intelligence · Autonomy · Trustworthiness · Reliability · Space

---

S. Straube (✉) · N. Will
Robotics Innovation Center, Deutsches Forschungszentrum für Künstliche Intelligenz GmbH (DFKI), Bremen, Germany
e-mail: sirko.straube@dfki.de; niels.will@dfki.de

N. Hoyer · F. Kirchner
Robotics Innovation Center, Deutsches Forschungszentrum für Künstliche Intelligenz GmbH (DFKI), Bremen, Germany
Robotics Research Group, University of Bremen, Bremen, Germany
e-mail: nina.hoyer@dfki.de; Frank.Kirchner@dfki.de

4.1 Results of Delphi Study

Population Survey: Research Questions, Results, and Explanation

The population survey examines the questions of how artificial intelligence (AI) will find its way into people's work and private lives and what acceptance such systems will meet in terms of application options in people's everyday lives.

The survey reveals that robots and AI are generally seen as thoroughly positive. Only 20% of respondents had a negative view of these two topics. Furthermore, the proportion of people who doubt the necessity of robots for society is only less than 10%. Accordingly, a high degree of willingness to accept robots can be assumed among the population.

Nevertheless, a deeper look into these topics shows that this result must be considered critically when it comes to *"reliability of systems"* and their *"areas of application."* On the first point *reliability of systems* only every third to fourth person surveyed considers robotic systems and AI to be reliable and error-free systems at the present time (for humans, safe and trustworthy technologies). However, when it comes to the need for robotic systems and AI regarding work that is too difficult or too dangerous for humans, the use is considered very likely. The more specific question on areas of application confirmed this result of the survey and showed very clearly that the acceptance of AI is depending on the area of application. By contrast, the use of robotic systems in the home environment or in the care of people is approached much more critically than the use of these technologies in the areas of space and deep-sea research.

This result is also reflected in the following questions of the representative survey: *"In which areas should robots be used as a priority?"* and *"In which areas should robots not be used at all?"*

The answers were given to the respondents in the form of a list of areas, so that a limited but covered answer option was already provided that addressed all areas of the study. Respondents were given the option of selecting up to five areas from this list: Industry, commercial, service sector, private life, medicine, human care, education, search and rescue, space exploration, marine/deep-sea exploration, transportation/logistics, agriculture, military, or in no field.

The evaluation showed that the respondents see the use of robots in the areas of space and deep-sea research predominantly in second and third place in percentage terms. Similarly, the area of search and rescue was seen as highly ranked (Fig. 4.1). In contrast, respondents had difficulty imagining the use of robots in the areas of human care (Fig. 4.2). In this ranking, areas of space and deep-sea research were not mentioned by respondents at all. Accordingly, areas that are rather distant and foreign to humans in general, both thematically and in terms of habitat.

The first question that arises here is how these preferences may occur among the population. One fundamental point could be the "distance" factor of the operational area. For many people surveyed, the areas of space and the deep-sea represent a field of application that seems distant and very abstract. It does not touch everyday life and is inaccessible to the public. The area of home care, however, represents a very

Rank 1	%	Rank 2	%	Rank 3	%	Rank 4	%	Rank 5	%
industry	28								
rescue	16	deep-sea	26						
space	16	space	15	space	22				
manufact.	10	industry	15	deep-sea	19	space	15		
deep-sea	10	healthcare	13	industry	16	healthcare	13	transport	16
		manufact.	10	rescue	13	industry	13	space	14
				healthcare	9	deep-sea	12	industry	10
						manufact.	11	agriculture	9
								military	9

Fig. 4.1 Priority preference ranking of application area of robot

Rank 1	%	Rank 2	%	Rank 3	%	Rank 4	%	Rank 5	%
care	27								
military	24	care	23						
privatelives	19	education	18	education	20				
No area	9	privatelives	15	leisure	20	privatelives	25		
leisure	9	service	12	care	14	education	25	leisure	22
		leisure	9	privatelives	13	service	13	care	21
				military	10	agriculture	11	education	13
						care	10	rescue	11
								service	11

Fig. 4.2 Ranking of non-preferred application area of robots

sensible application area people have personal associations with. In addition, there is the factor of "empathy" or "emotions," which is generally not associated with a robotic system—a machine. In distant places of application, the latter factor is not considered. Here, the inaccessibility and the safety of the human being are in the foreground.

Based on the current state of general knowledge within the population, the use of robotic systems in challenging and hostile environments instead of areas in everyday life is therefore a reasonable conclusion. We will take this favoured application field here and take a closer look what exactly robots have to be capable of when operating in deep-sea or space and how this relates to a robot being perceived as an autonomous system. The results may give answers why the survey results have shown that currently respondents do not trust robotic systems well enough to let them operate in sensitive environments for humans, e.g., in the care domain.

Potential Mission Scenarios of Robotic Systems in Harsh Environments

A potential field of hostile application area for robotic systems is the exploration of planetary surfaces (see Fig. 4.3). In this possible mission scenario, different robotic systems work together on a defined task as a team. Systems with a longer range can explore the environment with the help of sensors and cameras and send more agile systems into areas to examine the environment in detail (Brinkmann et al., 2019). Different means of transportation can also be an advantage here due to the different undergrounds and strengths, so that some tasks can only be completed successfully

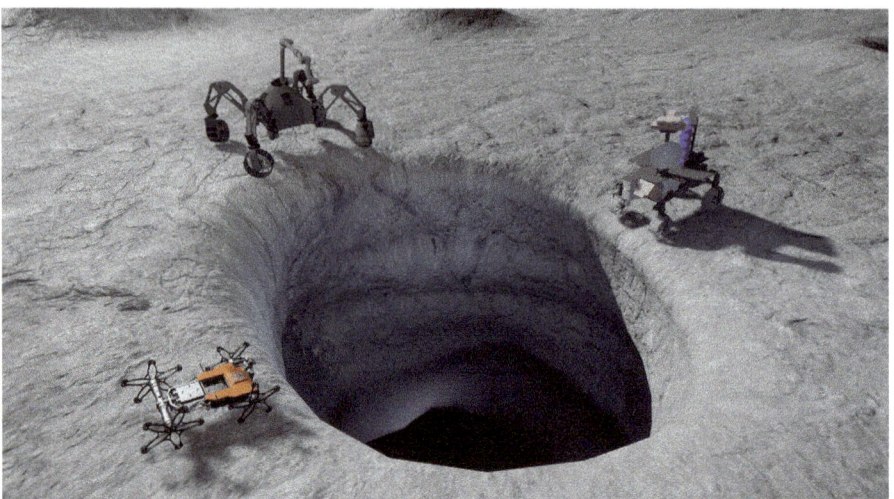

Fig. 4.3 Cooperative robotic team mission—Exploration of extraterrestrial planetary surfaces (Source: DFKI GmbH, Finn Lichtenberg)

in a team. Furthermore, systems with grippers can take ground samples and pass them to other systems for conservation. Another possible mission is the exploration of caves. Here, robotic systems can be lowered into these caves by other systems and the environment can be explored by cameras.

In addition to extraterrestrial environments, the deep-sea on Earth is also an area of operation that represents a hostile and hardly accessible environment for humans (see Fig. 4.4). Here, in addition to the inspection and maintenance of infrastructures located on the seabed (cables, pipelines, offshore installations), the focus is also on the exploration of new areas that have not yet been discovered and/or are not accessible to humans, and thus on the research and answering of wide-ranging scientific questions. Robotic systems equipped with sensors can take over these tasks for humans or support them in their tasks.[1]

Other examples represent the use of robotic systems in disaster areas to assist in human rescue and recovery, e.g., burial/collapse of buildings (Queralta et al., 2020). In this case, it is possible to drive camera-equipped robotic systems into areas that are difficult or impossible for humans to access in order to find potential victims, gain a general overview of the situation, and rescue them in the further progress. This avoids that human have to enter dangerous areas without knowing if there are people to be rescued in this area.

To use robots effectively in these or similar applications in the future, a clarity and a definition of the level of required and desired autonomy is necessary. This also shapes the required interaction with a human and our understanding of robots and humans working together. Mission operations in hostile environments—in space, in

---

[1] https://robotik.dfki-bremen.de/de/forschung/robotersysteme/flatfish/ (accessed on 14/01/2022).

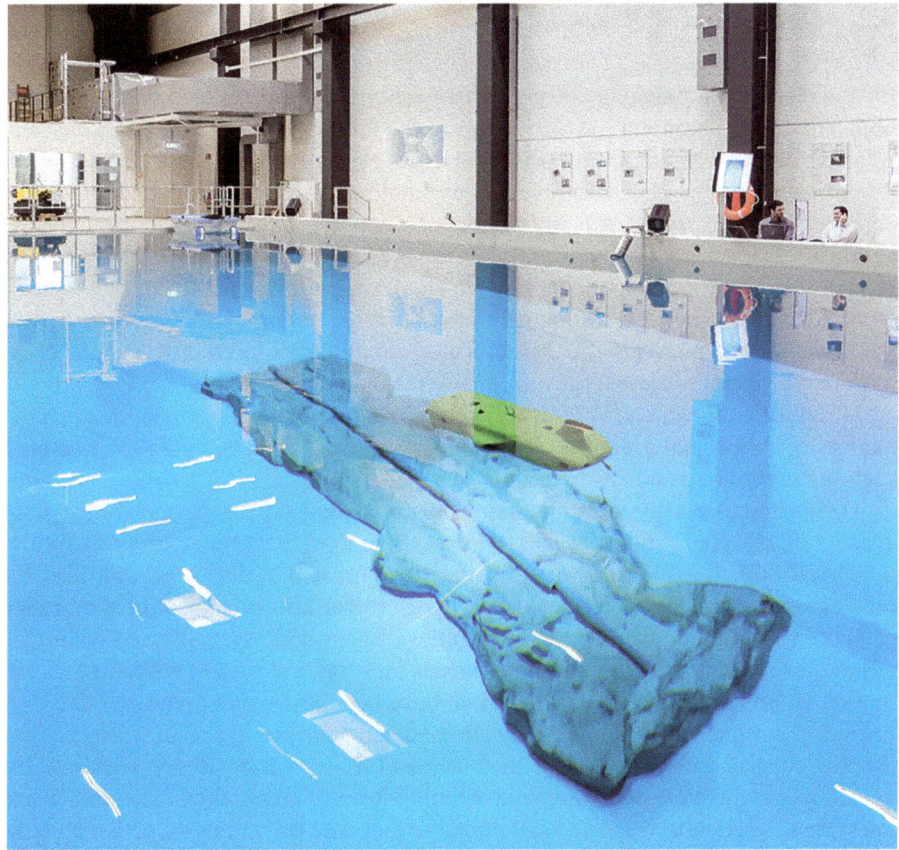

Fig. 4.4 Mission scenario of a pipeline inspection mission (Source: DFKI GmbH, Jan Albiez)

the deep-sea, or in hard-to-reach or existing catastrophic areas—are challenging and expose humans to significant hazards and risks. Robotic systems with high autonomy capabilities can help humans to reduce potential hazards and risks in a wide variety of situations. Furthermore, with the help of these systems, it is possible to explore or gain access to environments that were or still are inaccessible.

In addition to hostile environments, a growing number of robotic systems are finding their way into people's everyday lives. In this case, it must be ensured that humans are supported in their activities and that any potential risk must be always ruled out.

In both cases, hostile environments and everyday lives scenarios, the degree of autonomy of a system can vary greatly depending on its use and task, as can the degree of human–robot interaction. A good work distribution is thus the essential requirement for successful cooperation between the system and the human.

4.2 Definition of Autonomy

First, a clear distinction must be given between the terms of autonomy and automation. The term "autonomy" is derived from the Greek (autonomia) and means *self-reliance* or *independence*. In various disciplines and subject areas, the term has different definitions. For example, in psychology and philosophy, autonomy is described as *"the ability of people to possess free will and make self-determining decisions"*.[2] In the case of a state, this means that it is able to make its own laws, govern itself, and make political decisions without interference from other states. Within a state, if an organization can function itself according to established rules, then it is autonomous (Dietz, 2013). Thus, "autonomy" refers to the right of an individual, group, or state to govern its own circumstances.

In robotics, there are a wide variety of approaches and models to define the term autonomy clearly and according to the underlying task and context in each case—a unifying definition is however still missing.

To illustrate how the term autonomy is depending on the perspective and the context of the application, let us take the example of a manufacturing facility in which robotic systems perform predefined automated tasks. E.g., consider the placing of an object on a conveyor belt by a gripper arm of a robot or the driving of platforms along predefined transport routes. The robotic systems used within the system do not make any decisions themselves. They are precise reproductions of motion and manufacturing sequences that have been tested and optimized to a high degree. Consequently, this is a highly automated manufacturing process. Now, if the process is changed slightly such that interactions with humans are required, the situation is completely changing, and a certain level of autonomy is required. Then, the systems used must respond to incoming sensor data and interact together with the human in an intelligent way to anticipate and react to actions and offer possible solutions to the human. Autonomous action would thus require decisions in individual situations for which these automated processes are not created. Such individual decision makings based on many factors that cannot be automated unify the existing definitions of autonomy and the variations and uncertainty that an autonomous robot has to deal with, come from the environment that could consist of simply the operation area, other robots or humans. Clearly, interaction with humans is among the highest challenges on autonomy of robotic systems, but in any case a clear distinction must be made between the activity (sequence of defined tasks) and the behavior (autonomous decision) of the system.

The successful distribution of work within a team of autonomous agents (AI agents, robots, humans) is also dependent on the respective application context. Every situation has different influences and depends on many factors, which can also change during an action, resulting in very diverse requirements regarding the autonomy of a system.

---

[2] https://psychologie.stangl.eu/definition/Autonomie.shtml (accessed on 04/01/2022).

Robotic systems can be classified according to their underlying level of autonomy. In general, a distinction is made between *non-autonomous* (teleoperated, controlled) and fully *autonomous systems*, although there are different degrees of autonomy within these categories (Kunze et al., 2018). This depends on the already mentioned requirement and complexity of the task to be fulfilled by the system. A fully autonomous system must have the competence to adapt its own action to the environment, the involved further systems, and/or humans, always with respect to the situation and to plan, replan, and react adequately to occurring change. All these actions must be highly dynamic and realizable in real time. This poses an enormous challenge to the system.

Based on this, most of the missions currently taking place involve a human being who is supported in his tasks with the help of the systems. This applies to missions in hostile environments as well as in everyday situations. These are typically teleoperation systems, which means that the robotic system carries out a task controlled by the human. By means of different communication channels, the system receives task and actions, thus enables the human to perform the task from a safe distance.

Fully autonomous systems, on the other hand, perform their tasks independently based on stated goals. This means that despite changes within the context, they find possible solutions and can make decisions—without the involvement of humans (Yanco & Drury, 2004; Endsley & Kaber, 1999).

Accordingly, autonomous systems are systems that have the ability and properties to independently achieve a task or goal(s) specified by humans without requiring human intervention within the selected solution path. The basis for this is that the system understands itself in its context via sensors and can respond to unpredictable situations based on given learning algorithms and react if necessary, so that the task or goal is still achieved.

4.3 Robots in Harsh Environments: Space and Underwater

Robotics and AI in General

Modern robotics can be interpreted as an embodiment of AI. Very high standards apply here, as systems must often rapidly interact with and behave in the world. This makes robotics an integrator for AI and certainly a field that integrates additional disciplines as well: Robots have a body with certain design, mechanics, and electronics, sensors and actuators, data flows and software programs that link it all together so that robots can interact with their environment.

Some examples of robots have already arrived in our everyday lives, as there are already product-ready systems that can be used for everyday applications. There are various examples, such as the robot as a lawn mower, vacuum cleaner, or mopping robot. The first systems that came onto the market here still had very little AI on board, if any at all. Take the lawn mowing robot, for example: there, the first solutions were such that the robot drove up to a signal wire, then performed a random rotation and continued driving until it arrived at the signal wire again. With this the job can be done, but this is pure heuristics and there is no decision, planning, or similar on the system. The result is also high inefficiency. On today's systems, however, market-ready AI processes have already been implemented, because these robots already create maps, make plans, and then travel along paths that they have planned beforehand.

Robots are also very present in research and development—in their own right, major advances are being made in many sub-disciplines of robotics. Currently, it is very exciting to deal with AI and this can be seen in many new developments, which can be found in the technical literature but also throughout the Internet, although in the latter the borderline between true new advancements and faked information to yield a higher public attention is blurred. Therefore, it is always strongly recommended to take a closer look to understand what the advertised progress really is.

The capabilities and the degree of autonomy that a robot has, depends very much on two factors: the intelligence of the design of the robot and the intelligence level that the algorithms provide. Much progress in the capabilities of algorithms has been made in the last years, mostly driven by the fact that increasingly complex (and deep) neural network classifiers could be constructed using most recent advances in computing hard- and software. Whenever these networks had access to huge amounts of examples, they could find patterns in the data that enabled them to classify new examples with a very high success rate. The public breakthrough here was the AlphaGo algorithm, which used deep neural networks and beat professional human Go players. In a prominent study published in 2017 (Silver et al., 2017), the authors were able to show that one can find other interesting properties in the AlphaGo algorithm: the algorithm was studied again and trained in different ways. Two examples can be mentioned here: In one case, the algorithm has been trained using data from human players and has learned to play the game based on these moves. In the other case, the algorithm was trained with a reinforcement learning algorithm that needed a bit more training time to achieve the same quality. The latter did not use rules, but the program received feedback on the completed moves in the form of a reward function. The interesting thing here is that this algorithm never saw a human player move before and learned to play the game purely based on the reward function. Looking at how well these algorithms predict the play of a human player, it was shown that the reinforcement learning algorithm can actually predict this function only with progressive training time on human player moves, although it was already able to play with comparable or better performance than a human before.

This means that today's AI procedures can develop their own strategies without any expert knowledge having been explicitly programmed in there, and not even the expert knowledge has been added via training examples. The complexity of the processes, for example, by building artificial neural networks with many layers, enables the systems to achieve the same performance as a human through trial and error, as in the example of the Go game. The advances in these algorithms have motivated major IT hardware companies, like Intel or NVIDIA, to develop specific boards as platforms for neural networks. E.g., NVIDIA used the popular domain of autonomous driving to demonstrate very catchily in the same year as the study from Silver et al. that one can already control vehicles with these artificial deep neural networks in many situations.[3]

These are first steps that show that technical solutions exist in rudiments that allow AI and robotics to move in our environment. They are impressive examples, but at the same time, there are many issues to be resolved before we can deploy these technologies. We also need to look at many factors when assessing the maturity of the technology, such as the extent to which algorithms can be deceived or manipulated. Staying with the example of autonomous driving, as with human drivers, errors will always occur with technical systems. This is also due to the environment in which decisions sometimes have to be made despite impaired vision (or technically ambiguous sensor data). Since the decision-making basis of an artificial neural network today is in the network itself (i.e., in the connection strength of individual neurons), the transparency of the AI is naturally lost as a result. Given the complexity of today's networks, this information is not easy to extract—but that is exactly what should happen. It is therefore very important in current research not only to enable systems to perform very complex actions, but also to develop mechanisms that make it possible to understand why an algorithm has made certain decisions and on what basis. The answers to these and other questions are already the subject of current research and will become even more important for the use of AI and robotics in the future.

Autonomy Helps When Uncertainty Is High: Requirements and Applications from Harsh Environments

When a robot should perform a mission in an unknown environment, e.g., in the context of space exploration on the moon or even on Mars, it will get into situations where standard procedures will not work. Then the robot either has to wait for external input (i.e., a human steering the robot) or, equipped with a certain level of intelligence, the robot could use the own sensor data and evaluate the available set of actions in order to choose an appropriate solution to solve the task and not violate any constraints. If the latter would actually happen, we would speak of an autonomous system (within a specified range or set of actions), which would be able to handle a certain level of complex situations. To achieve this, robots would need to have the capability too generally be able to sense and interpret their environment, and thus make plans for how to act and/or move in that environment. On top of this ability would ideally come capabilities that would qualify robots for a natural interaction with humans, be it through communication with a human located somewhere else (e.g., robot on the moon, human on the earth) or that humans are working directly together with robots on-site for a certain task. Robots then need to have capabilities for speech recognition, understanding, and speech generation. In addition, the ability to learn is important as well, so that the robots can improve in their performance—for this they must be able to evaluate their own actions and learn from

---

[3] see https://www.youtube.com/watch?v=-96BEoXJMs0&t for an illustration.

mistakes. Therefore, this is ultimately the idea of the robot in the future: it is no longer purely about automating processes, but about systems that basically move in their environment with an ability to make their own decisions and interact flexibly with it, as well as with other robots or humans.

The autonomy capabilities discussed above can be very useful for robots exploring the solar system and probably also exploiting extraterrestrial resources. In this regard, robots can perform tasks that play a major role in extraterrestrial missions here in the future by developing various new features. These include exploring surfaces, searching for life, understanding how the solar system was formed, and also finding new resources. For the robots, this means they must be able to reliably sample with high robustness, explore, perform analysis, and then also return to stations where they can upload and share their data. Robots can also be used for longer human stays on extraterrestrial surfaces, and they will also play a strong role in the future for work directly with or near humans. In particular, they can be used to mine and utilize resources directly on site, e.g., not to transport all construction materials to other planets, as this would drastically increase mission costs. Instead, resources can be used on site, robots can help or provide the construction of extraterrestrial structures, as well as assembly and also maintenance work of these infrastructures. For all these tasks, autonomy is very important—in the following, we use examples from three potential targets for space missions and their specific characteristics: the Moon, Mars, and Jupiter's Moon Europa. These examples will be used to show what requirements for robotics are important and will play a role in the future.

On the earth's satellite, the moon, there are craters in polar regions that can be explored and used, and there are caves that may also offer possibilities as habitats and could be of importance for the establishment of a moon base. This idea could be approached and perhaps realized with autonomous robots. To make the moon usable by space travel and in turn to use it as a stopover for further space missions has long been a dream of mankind. For missions on the moon, robots are primarily a way to clearly keep the costs of realizing this dream under control and to keep the infrastructures technically functional even without the presence of humans. On the next destination, Mars, there are many more hurdles for space missions: flights to Mars take longer than a year, communication has such high hurdles that controlling a complex operation becomes almost impossible and takes an enormous amount of time. On Mars, there is also the exploration of the surfaces, the mapping, sampling, and search for information on the formation up to the search for life as the first use case, which is already operated by the first systems. These systems have partly autonomous functions, but they are not autonomous even in their exploration movements, but completely controlled. There are craters on Mars in whose sediment layers water or ice is suspected under certain circumstances. In addition, there are regions on Mars, such as the Valles Marineris valley system, which seem to be interesting for building infrastructures there as well and possibly then being able to establish a base or infrastructure on Mars in the distant future. Here, too, autonomous robots can be used to maintain such infrastructures.

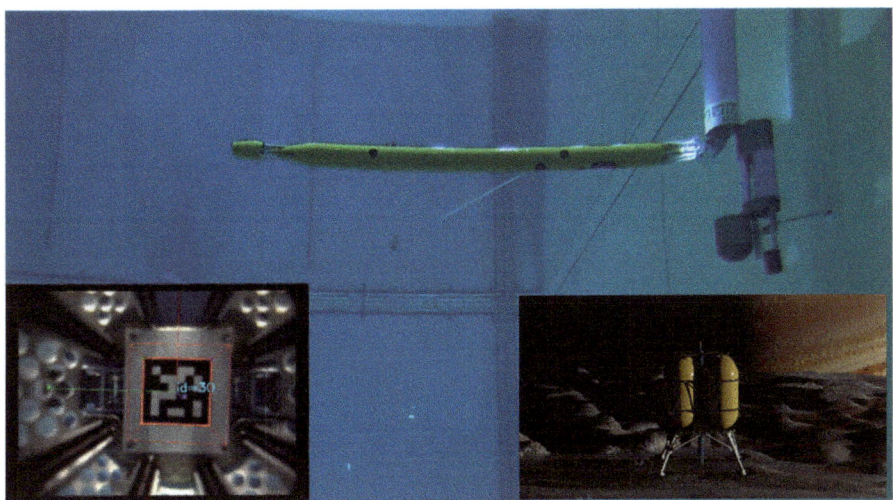

Fig. 4.5 Docking experiment in the Leng robot maritime exploration hall for exploration of Jupiter's moon Europa. Camera image bottom left, rendering of a Europa moon probe bottom right. (Source: DFKI GmbH)

A very special example of requirements for autonomous systems is provided by the even more distant moon of Jupiter, Europa. Here, under a thick layer of ice, an ocean of up to 100 km depth is suspected. To explore its seafloor in search of extraterrestrial life, autonomous underwater robots are ultimately needed that, after landing a probe and subsequently penetrating the ice layer, are able to carry out autonomous exploration missions with little energy consumption and can deliver the data back to the probe accordingly. As a study for such a mission, the Leng robot[4] was developed together with other mission components (Hildebrandt et al., 2013). The robot is shaped to fit into a possible ice drill, navigates autonomously, and is capable of diving passively (without energy consumption) to then actively explore on the seafloor. Upon return, the robot can perform autonomous docking for data transfer (see Fig. 4.5).

Just like in the space domain, robots operating in the deep-sea need AI desperately for autonomous operations, since communication is very difficult and unforeseen occurrences (like changes in currents) are likely (for a comprehensive overview on challenges and technologies, see Kirchner et al. (2020)).

Autonomy: Insights from Field Tests

A good illustration of the current state of the art for autonomous robots is to look at the setup, results, and tasks from field tests, especially in the space domain. Here, multinational teams of research institutions and companies come together to test, evaluate, and at best fulfill a given mission scenario. Such field tests also show how

---

[4]https://robotik.dfki-bremen.de/de/forschung/robotersysteme/leng/ (accessed on 14/01/2022).

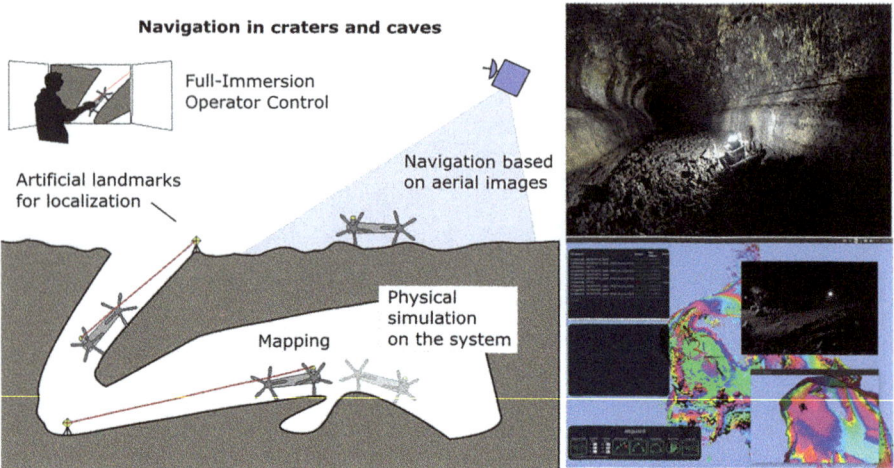

Fig. 4.6 Analog mission: Exploration of caves on the island of Tenerife—the robot captures its environment, plans and simulates the next steps before final execution. (Source: DFKI GmbH)

the interaction of all components works, i.e., in most cases how mobility, manipulation, and also navigation capabilities work together to achieve the specific goal. One example is the exploration of lava caves on the island of Tenerife, as an analogue environment for corresponding caves on the Moon or Mars (Schwendner et al., 2015), as illustrated in Fig. 4.6. The robots explored these caves, and multiple systems also used a common representation of this environment and mapped it further. The robots themselves generated landmarks to orient themselves. As exploration has progressed, simulation of next steps has taken place directly on the system to verify them. Thus, the robots have been autonomous in the caves, planning their action, simulating it, then executing it, and mapping the caves accordingly on their own. Here, the robot has a high mobility by design and the capability for navigation in the caves. Still, many capabilities are missing, if troubles would be encountered, e.g., if the way back would be blocked somehow or sensors would fail or be wrong. Such kind of self-monitoring and also reasoning about the current status is still not realized in systems qualified for such field tests.

Another scenario in the field is exploration as a team of robots with different morphologies and capabilities, e.g., a bigger supply robot in combination with a small scouting unit. Likewise, the scenario depicted in Fig. 4.7 is showing a field test performed in the desert of Utah in North America with the Sherpa TT robot, which carried various mission modules, and the Coyote III robot, which was equipped with a small arm to take samples and also explore (Sonsalla et al., 2017; Cordes et al., 2018). The two robots successfully completed their mission in a period of 6 weeks. Part of the test, in addition to pure cooperation within the robot team, was interaction with a human, who used an exoskeleton to teleoperate the Sherpa TT in particularly difficult situations. This type of field test brings the systems closer to the real

4 The Challenge of Autonomy: What We Can Learn from Research on...

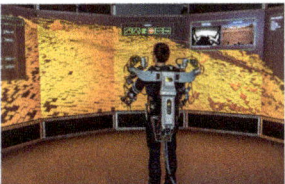
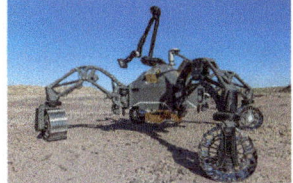
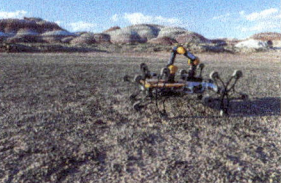

Mission Control in Bremen with Exo-Skeleton *SherpaTT* – equipped with P/L-Items and BaseCamp *Coyote III* and *SIMA* manipulation arm

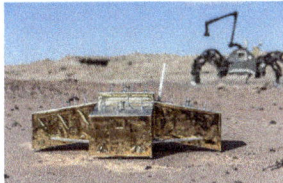
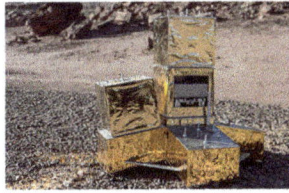
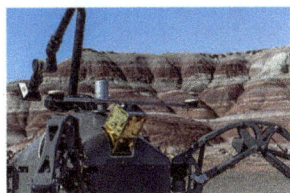

BaseCamp with 5 electro-mechanical interfaces *BaseCamp* with 3 *P/L-Items* connected *DGPS module* connected to SherpaTT

Fig. 4.7 Elements from the field test in Utah—The robot team consists of the robot Sherpa (top center) and the small rover Coyote III (top right). In special situations, the systems are addressed via teleoperation supported by an exoskeleton (top left). (Source: DFKI GmbH)

conditions that will be used later and also provides the scientists with a whole range of experience in the appropriate use of the systems. Again, the robots could cooperate and solve the task, but also a well-designed interface for teleoperation was necessary (Planthaber et al., 2017). This illustrated that humans are in most processes inevitable giving their inputs and helping the robots out of situations where these are lost. Therefore, a cooperative task solving in a mixture of robots and humans (be it distant or on-site) is currently still one of the best approaches for complex missions with robots. As already mentioned in the beginning, the better the interaction capabilities of robots become (e.g., for reporting problems or errors), the more efficient will a task be handled.

Task Sharing Between Humans and Robots
In the future, it will not only be a matter of sending autonomous robots alone into space or to extraterrestrial planets to have them autonomously carry out missions there, but it will also be a matter of having robots act together with humans. This topic is not only relevant in space robotics, but also central to the further development applications for rehabilitation or production purposes (e.g., in Industry 4.0), being areas in the Delphi survey where respondents were more skeptical with integration of robots. One immediate application for robots in space would be to perform on-orbit servicing, for example, to remove space debris from orbit, or to perform maintenance and support work on satellites or the International Space Station (ISS).

Task sharing could occur on very different interaction levels with the extremes of teleoperation on one side and full autonomy on the other. In the simplest case, a robot can be controlled directly, which then does nothing independently, but basically carries out the actions specified by the human. The more immersive the teleoperation is, the better is the human situated in the situation of the robot and

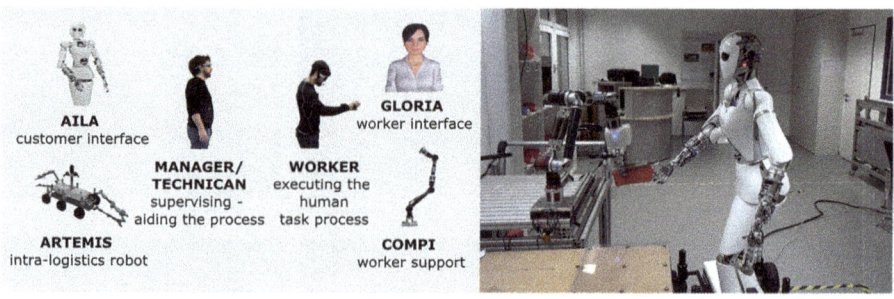

Fig. 4.8 Example of a hybrid team with possible roles (left) and recordings of autonomous robot–robot interaction (right). (Source: DFKI GmbH)

the better can the human react as if being the robot. In addition to pure teleoperation, humans can order commands to robots, which are then executed. These commands can occur on subtask level ("drive straight") or even include objects in the scenario ("drive to the door") and the granularity depends on what the robot is capable of understanding about its environment and the won capabilities. Typically, such commands are elicited by explicit forms of interaction, such as through speech and gestures, but implicit interaction interfaces are also possible, e.g., by directly recording data from humans using eye tracking, or muscle or neurophysiological data and integrating it into the interaction with a robot. Through this, information can already be collected in prediction of whether certain movements will be executed by the person, which can then be more quickly recorded by the system and also translated or supported. Also, via the evaluation of neurophysiological data it can be determined in principle whether an overload of the human being is currently present and thus under certain circumstances information is available which has not yet been perceived and processed by the human being, or vice versa: perceived but currently classified as unimportant. When developing robotic systems for direct interaction, it is most important to build systems that are very compliant and thus largely harmless and safe to humans.

An important, overriding topic in the interaction of humans and robots, which is, however, still far away from real use in space missions, is the formation of the so-called hybrid teams of humans and robots (see Fig. 4.8). This involves close cooperation between humans, robots, and also virtual agents or other AI systems in a team structure (Schwartz et al., 2016). The robot continues to be an assistant for the human, but it should behave so independently that it is also perceived by the human as a team partner. This means that a robot can independently take over and complete work without having to be given complete instructions. Work in hybrid teams is supported by planning algorithms in the background. Technologies must also be developed and integrated that are robustly capable of recognizing human intuitions and making them available digitally. Digital agents, in turn, which are available to humans via voice input, help to provide humans with direct information from the digital representation.

For a team of humans and robots, a functioning interaction with each other applies in all cases, e.g. autonomous handovers of workpieces must be successfully carried out with each other and also negotiated. For example, when all members of a team are acting in a highly autonomous manner, such handoffs cannot simply be programmed in, but the systems need heuristics and protocols according to which they can negotiate and perform such handoffs autonomously. Then such teams could perform joint assembly or joint infrastructure construction on an extraterrestrial surface.

4.4 Robots Supporting in Everyday Life

Today, robots are no longer exclusively found in factories. Robotic systems, or at least robot components, can already be found in everyday technical systems such as cars, tools, or home products. One growing target area of application are robots for everyday support and services: Robots should help to improve the quality of life and increasingly operate in contexts in which only humans previously acted. This applies to both the professional (e.g., in manufacturing companies) and the private sector (e.g., household). The motivation for this is to reduce physically strenuous activities, monotonous stresses, and strains. Even in view of demographic change—people want to live independently in their familiar surroundings as long as possible—robotic systems become increasingly relevant. However, it is also obvious that as soon as a complex robotic system is leaving a controlled environment—such as a production hall—challenges arise in terms of safe, economically, and efficient use, that can only be mastered in an interdisciplinary approach and must consider ethical, legal, and social implications beyond technical issues.

An ideal autonomous system for everyday life scenarios must be able to act independently, learn, solve complex tasks, and react to unpredictable events. Thus, to provide safe and meaningful support in everyday life, it is expected that human abilities and characteristics in various areas are transferable to the technical system. But safe movement over obstacles is only one part of the challenge. The reason for this is that people on the street, at home, in the supermarket or comparable everyday situations often move unpredictably. According to that, a domestic robot that takes over a variety of household tasks, such as tidying up, cleaning, and setting the table, must work very reliably and must have reliable sensors in order to damage something or—in the worst case, to hurt people. However, the safe everyday use of such multifunctional and complex systems is still a future scenario. The effort and costs for a step into everyday life use is currently a too strong barrier in relation to the benefits. The previously presented results from the population survey show that this is also part of the public perspective. Only every third to fourth person surveyed considers robotic systems and AI to be reliable and error-free systems at the present time. On the other hand, market figures from the HEMIX (Home Electronics Market

Index), a joint project of gfu and GfK,[5] show that consumers in Germany are increasingly counting on robots to help with household tasks. Around 620.000 household robots were sold in Germany in the first half of 2021, an increase of 6%. This relates to vacuum cleaning robots, lawn mowing robots, and window cleaning robots. Therefore, at least for special applications, the everyday use of robots is already practicable today. As the exploration of lava caves on the island of Tenerife shows, the complex navigation capabilities of robot systems are one of the basic skills for autonomous robots in harsh environments. This also applies to domestic robots. Today, for example, vacuum cleaner robots map their surroundings instead of driving randomly through an apartment. They are equipped with cameras and object recognition and thus perform their tasks much better and more reliably than just a few years ago. Furthermore, such systems are becoming more and more affordable.

Moreover, in other areas of application, such as care, it is not to be expected soon that humanoid robots with a wide range of capabilities will be used, but rather learning assistance systems specialized for a specific task. The systems used in rehabilitation medicine can be divided into different application areas. On the one hand, systems are designed that are used for the motor recovery of patients and, on the other hand, robotic assistance systems are designed to support the everyday actions of affected patients and to assist nursing care tasks. These include, for example, intelligent wheelchairs with robotic gripping aids or service robots. Another group is social robotics, which is used for entertainment or to simulate closeness to living beings.

The use of intelligent assistance systems is intended to relieve the burden on nursing staff and at the same time helping care recipients to become more independent. Systems are designed, e.g., to support caregivers and patients in everyday, physically demanding care activities on the nursing bed (Hawes et al., 2017).

For this purpose, for example, an adaptive and multifunctional motorized bed with a robotic arm system for use in care is being developed.[6] Sensor components are used to be able to adjust the bed position depending on the situation. Various holding and support functions of the robot arm are indented, for example, for bed-wheelchair transfer. The system is also intended to continuously monitor the posture of the nurses during the mobilization or transfer of care recipients and to provide guidance on optimization in the event of unfavorable loads. A partially automated bed-robot arm system can improve the autonomy and quality of life of care recipients. For carers, robotic support for lifting and moving a patient can represent a significant reduction in physical stress. This prevents damage or diseases of the lower back area.

Efforts to integrate robotic systems into care are also based on expanding therapeutic options, enabling patients to do more of their own training and relieving the burden on therapists. For example, intelligent exoskeletons are being designed and used for robotic rehabilitation of neurological disorders.

---

[5] https://gfu.de/markt-zahlen/hemix-2021/ (accessed on 10/01/2022).

[6] https://adamekor.de (accessed on 10/01/2022).

As a robotic system, the exoskeleton represents, in simple terms, an external support structure which is directly connected to the human body and is as an active system equipped with actuators and sensors. This results in a wide range of interaction possibilities in the context of rehabilitation between the exoskeleton and the human users of the system. An exoskeleton usually has several contact points to the human body. This specific structure makes it possible to guide and stabilize the patient's arm at each joint and to implement a high number of active degrees of freedom to realize finely coordinated movement patterns. The active stabilization of the limb by the exoskeleton enables the compensation of the inherent weight of the system and the weight of the limb and allows training under the exclusion of "gravity," as well as the passive movement guidance of the limb even without the patient's own effort, if necessary (Kumar et al., 2019). The aim is to create in an intelligent way synergies between man and machine to optimize processes and the workflow of rehabilitation, as well as to provide patients and therapists with advanced and innovative therapy options on the basis of this new technology.

In summary, in contrast to classical industrial robots, where the operating conditions can be controlled very well, robots in everyday human life must be able to adapt to the constantly changing environment. This implies high demands on the hardware and the software and results in a high complexity of intelligent robot systems. The high complexity results among others from the dependencies between the individual components. One example of this is the number of degrees of freedom and sensors, as well as their arrangement and the number of incoming data/information in interaction with the software and control components. Therefore, it is expected that we see in near future more semi-autonomous systems in everyday use, which can carry out low-threshold functions independently such as independently driving around obstacles or avoiding collisions when handing over objects. For the time being, complex decisions and activities will still be left to humans. It is also to be expected that initially specialized systems will find their way into everyday life, rather than generalized assistance robotics.

4.5 Competence for Autonomy

The applications described in the previous sections made already clear that full autonomy including informed decisions in an unknown and typically dynamic environment is currently hard to achieve—if not impossible—for a robot. Key components for autonomy are the knowledge of the own capabilities and the validation of taken actions with respect to the task, the environment, and the current situation. A fully autonomous system would have to know these parameters dynamically, while having the ability to respond to new and unforeseen events at any time. Instead of concentrating only on the final stage of full autonomy, certain levels of autonomy have been defined, e.g., in the car industry, to classify existing systems with respect to the required input from a human. A closer look at this approach reveals two problems: First, the step between the last but one level and the final level of full autonomy is in reality a big step including a mandatory self-awareness of the systems which is currently not achieved. Second, a system behaving in a natural environment may perform different tasks in different situations and may therefore request assistance in situation A while running fully autonomous in situation B. Due to this, it is more appropriate to not classify systems as fully autonomous or not, but to rather look at the functionality of the system with respect to the task to judge whether the system can fulfill the task autonomously or not. In their framework paper on robot autonomy levels in human–robot interaction (HRI), Beer et al. (2014) render this general conception of autonomy asking five central questions (they denote as guidelines):

1. What task is the robot going to perform? Here a classification of the relevant variables is made.
2. What aspects of the task should the robot perform? Here, subtasks are defined.
3. To what extent can the robot perform those aspects? Here, the amount of required human intervention is classified.
4. What level can the robot's autonomy be categorized? This typically responds to most autonomy classifications elsewhere ranging from full teleoperation over shared-control to full autonomy.
5. How might autonomy influence the HRI variables? Here, it is questioned to what extent the robot might be influenced (e.g., in learning), how the human might be influenced (e.g., in trust) and how the social relation between the two might change.

These questions illustrate that determining the right level of autonomy is depending on many factors which can also change over time (for an extensive discussion, see Beyerer et al. (2021)). The needed level of autonomy is depending on environment and type of task—this contrasts with capabilities of the system in combination with legal and ethical guidelines. A possible workflow how a task could be treated by an autonomous system is illustrated in Fig. 4.9, showing how complicated this process can get when problems occur. Repeatedly the system has to analyze its own state with respect to the task and the environment and compare this with execution criteria. In other words, the someone or the system itself has to evaluate its competence to handle the situation appropriately.

Therefore, a central issue for an autonomous system is the issue of competence and the limitations of the system. In each situation, one could ask the question: Does a given system have the competence to perform the task or not? Nowadays in nearly all situation we—the humans—judge about the competence of a robot or a machine, or—in case of other humans—we look at qualifications to estimate a competence. E.g., in a space mission, it is clearly ruled what the robot is allowed to perform on its own and where teleoperation is applied.

Now, if people think of robots (in particular in harsh environments), they often think of highly autonomous systems, i.e. of systems that can perform most of the tasks on their own. As has been outlined above, this means the occurrence of uncertainties in a complex environment that the robot has to deal with. A successful accomplishment of tasks or missions in such situations requires that the robot can

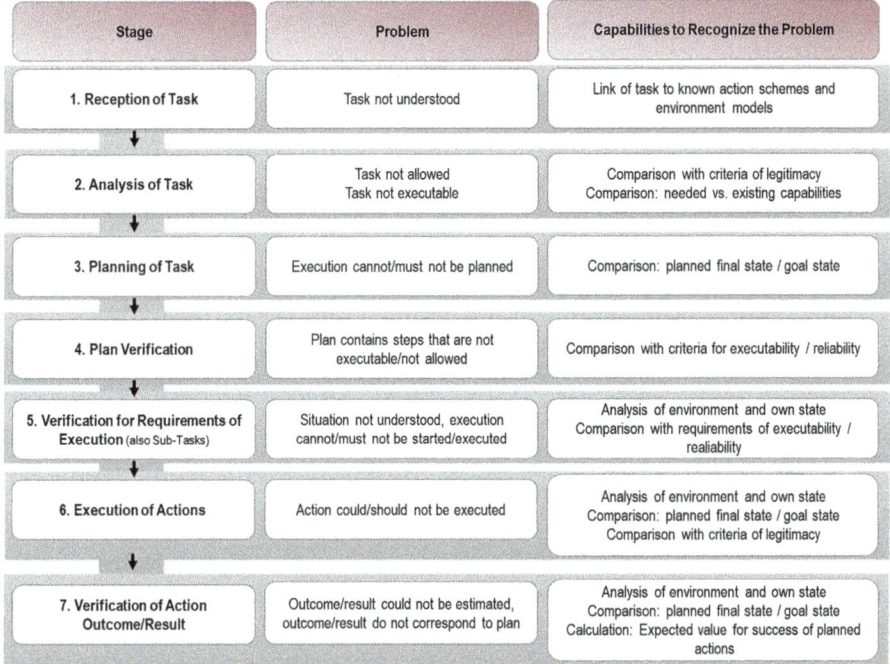

Fig. 4.9 Possible workflow for task execution of an autonomous system (after Beyerer et al. (2021), with permission of Plattform Lernende Systeme)

judge whether it can handle the situation on its own or if assistance is needed (from a human or another system). This judgement is a judgement of competence—and the systematic analysis of its own competence is hard to achieve for a robot, since no general formula is known and several areas of knowledge are required to be taken into account, where each area alone is a field of currently ongoing research: required and available capabilities, possible options for actions, and constraints to act (e.g., of legal or ethical nature). It is shown in Fig. 4.10 that while the mode of execution with respect to autonomy can be illustrated in a direct relationship, the judgement of competence for autonomy is a function which is depending on the values and the weights of the above-mentioned factors. It is therefore not straightforward to derive competence from one of these factors alone: A system can have few capabilities, but since it may have many options to act and nearly no further constraints, it might have enough competence to perform the task autonomously (green line in Fig. 4.10). Since such models are not existing in a complete form, today, this analysis is still typically done by qualified humans if robots should perform autonomous tasks in an unknown and/or dynamic environment. Alternatively, the complexity and power of the robot is reduced, so that more simplified systems (like a vacuum cleaning robot) perform only few well-defined tasks automatically without the danger of causing any harm to humans and the environment due to power and safety procedures. However, these robots do not establish trust by humans due to their sophisticated autonomy,

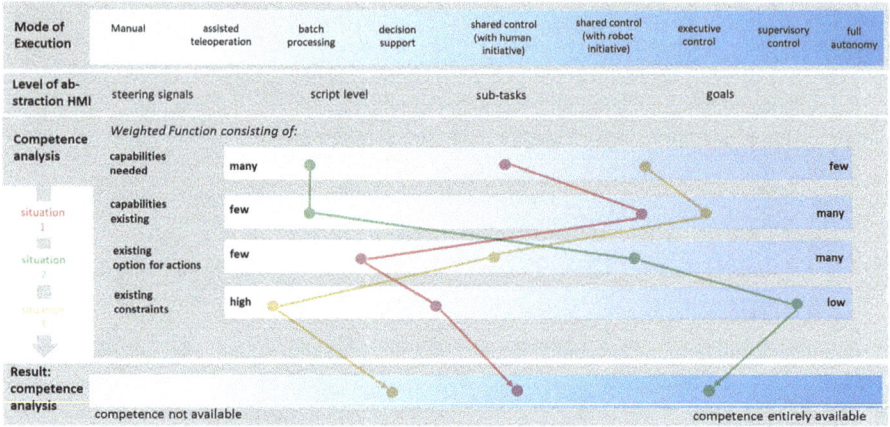

Fig. 4.10 A model for autonomy based on the dependency on competence (after Beyerer et al. (2021), with permission from Plattform Lernende Systeme)

but rather through their simplicity. This might be a reason, why people find it hard to imagine, how a more flexible and general autonomous robot would look like, and how communication would take place with such a system.

4.6 Conclusions: Establishing Trust Between Humans and Robots

Autonomy of machines is an old vision of humans, and the imagination how this might look like has been visualized and devised in drawings, animations, books, and films. Currently, we are crossing a border to really see robots and cars move and operate in our environment without direct human intervention, but what we see today still has many drawbacks and large discrepancies exist between today's reality and the stories and pictures in our minds. Many tasks that seem without effort for human beings are still impossible for robots, and still not understood by humans. Therefore, the underlying complexity is extremely high and research on AI and robotics often involves hardware/software co-design and not separated developments. Hardware is developed that must be controlled and thus co-defines the behavior of the systems, i.e., new hardware also means new possibilities in behavior. Often challenges also arise from multimodal sensor streams, which often have to be processed adaptively. Values in these sensors need to be identified and classified, because not everything the sensors pick up is important, but the important features relevant to the intended behavior need to be found. Robotics is also about planning, re-planning, executing, and adapting motion and action. Now, the more complex the system should behave, the more complex hardware and software will get, with, e.g., more and more actuators that ultimately all have to be controlled to trigger a behavior, as well as very high, partly parallel data streams, which have to be processed, possibly stored, and integrated. This must be aligned with various software levels working together up to a certain point that humans would classify as goal-directed behavior. It is because of this complexity level that no one really oversees how long it will take to really cross the border to have autonomous systems around and how human societies might change with such new technological advances.

The results of the study have indicated that the public view on robotics is generally positive, while at the same time people tend to favor robotic systems much stronger in application fields where no humans are nearby (e.g., in harsh environments) and not in fields where robots will directly act together with humans or also on humans (e.g., in the care domain). This shows that the greatest challenge is the still widespread lack of trust and the acceptance of people toward robotic systems—especially systems that occur in everyday life. It directly relates to our everyday experience that technical systems may fail in a systematic way without any visible explanation with—in terms of powerful systems—possibly severe consequences. Today's robots do not have sufficient capability to understand the context and relate this to the own set of available actions in the particular situation, and to give appropriate feedback and possibly also explanations to the human, e.g. if failure is occurring (which is always possible).

It is therefore worthwhile to take a look at the current research in domains where the autonomy of the robot is a crucial question for its successful application. Typically, these are harsh environments where humans cannot go or only under high efforts and taking large risks. The most prominent example in this chapter here is the important role of autonomous robots for future space missions in several scenarios. These scenarios require capabilities for the autonomous exploration of the extraterrestrial surfaces, also in a team of several robots, the construction of infrastructure, and the direct interaction of humans and robots, for example, via telemanipulation or also via concepts in which robots and humans interact with each other in a kind of team and carry out missions together.

For robots in terrestrial scenarios, similar questions regarding capabilities and autonomy have to be addressed. Examples exist from underwater robotics, where humans are still far away, up to industrial robotics where humans can in principle even share the workspace with the robot. And if the workspace is shared, many other fields of application exist as well, which can benefit from the development of the technologies and in turn also provide new impetus for space travel. Examples for applications with direct contact to humans would be the use of robots in rescue missions or robotic technology for rehabilitation, e.g., after stroke. For the latter, for example, parts of the exoskeleton technology can be used as intelligent robots built around humans to support the rehabilitation process. Even other domains that receive much attention at the moment, like the question of autonomous driving and new mobility concepts are also emerging as a result of the technologies discussed here.

It remains a major challenge to develop autonomous robots that are capable of relating task and context to the competence of own actions and ideally directly learn from the choices taken. This would be one technological basis to realize the vision of robots autonomously working together with humans. On top, it requires advances in safety and the transparency on decisions in order to establish trust with the humans—probably declared by elaborated certification mechanisms. Everywhere, where this is not (yet) possible, robotic systems will be limited in function and flexibility.

Robotics is thus a very interdisciplinary field. The combination of engineering sciences and computer science alone is not sufficient; other sciences must also be involved. The more you use mechanisms with high internal complexity, such as deep neural learning, the more you also need methods from other sciences, such as neuroscience, to develop methods for making systems transparent. Overall, it is in many cases a matter of dealing with increasing complexity, and that for systems that are supposed to be endowed with long-term autonomy. To enable them to operate on the moon or Mars, for example, the robots must function robustly and safely over a long period of time.

References

Beer, J., Fisk, A., & Rogers, W. (2014). Toward a framework for levels of robot autonomy in human-robot interaction. *Journal of Human-Robot Interaction, 3*(2), 74–99.

Beyerer J., Straube S., Deserno T., Tchouchenkov I., & Wedler A. (2021, Feb). Kompetent im Einsatz Variable Autonomie Lernender Systeme in lebensfeindlichen Umgebungen. *Lernende Systeme - Die Plattform für künstliche Intelligenz.*

Brinkmann, W., Cordes, F., Koch, C. E. S., Wirkus, M., Dominguez, R., Dettmann, A., Vögele, T., & Kirchner, F. (2019, November 19–21). Space robotic systems and artificial intelligence in the context of the European space technology roadmap. In *Proceedings of Space Tech Conferences, Bremen.*

Cordes, F., Kirchner, F., & Babu, A. (2018). Design and field testing of a rover with an actively articulated suspension system in a Mars analog terrain. *Journal of Field Robotics, 35*(7), 1149–1181.

Dietz, K. M. (2013). Die Entdeckung der Autonomie bei den Griechen. *Forum Classicum, 4*, 256.

Endsley, M. R., & Kaber, D. B. (1999). Level of automation effects on performance, situation awareness and workload in a dynamic control task. *Ergonomics, 42*(3), 462–492. https://doi.org/10.1080/001401399185595

Hawes, N., et al. (2017). The STRANDS project: Long-term autonomy in everyday environments. *IEEE Robotics & Automation Magazine, 24*(3), 146–156. https://doi.org/10.1109/MRA.2016.2636359

Hildebrandt, M., Albiez, J., Wirtz, M., Kloss, P., Hilljegerdes, J., & Kirchner, F. (2013, September 23). Design of an autonomous under-ice exploration system. In *MTS/IEEE Oceans 2013 San Diego, (OCEANS-2013), San Diego, CA* (pp. 1–6). IEEE.

Kirchner, F., Straube, S., Kühn, D., & Hoyer, N. (Eds.). (2020). *AI technology for underwater robots* (Vol. 96). Springer.

Kumar, S., Wöhrle, H., Trampler, M., Simnofske, M., Peters, H., Mallwitz, M., Kirchner, E. A., & Kirchner, F. (2019). Modular design and decentralized control of the recupera exoskeleton for stroke rehabilitation. *Applied Sciences, 9*(4), 626.

Kunze, L., Hawes, N., Duckett, T., Hanheide, M., & Krajnik, T. (2018). Artificial intelligence for long-term robot autonomy: A survey. *IEEE Robotics and Automation Letters, 3*(4), 4023–4030. https://doi.org/10.1109/LRA.2018.2860628

Planthaber, S., Maurus, M, Bongardt, B., Mallwitz, M., Vaca Benitez, L. M., Christensen, L., Cordes, F., Sonsalla, R., Stark, T., & Roehr, T. M. (2017, March 06–09). Controlling a semi-autonomous robot team from a virtual environment. In *Proceedings of the HRI conference, (HRI), Vienna.* ACM/IEEE.

Queralta, J. P., Taipalmaa, J., Pullinen, B. C., Sarker, V. K., Gia, T. N., Tenhunen, H., Gabbouj, M., Raitoharju, J., & Westerlund, T. (2020). Collaborative multi-robot search and rescue: Planning, coordination, perception, and active vision. *IEEE Access, 8,* 191617–191643. https://doi.org/10.1109/ACCESS.2020.3030190

Schwartz, T., Feld, M., Bürckert, C., Dimitrov, S., Folz, J., Hevesi, P., Hutter, D., Kiefer, B., Krieger, H. U., Lüth, C., Mronga, D., Pirkl, G., Spieldenner, T., Wirkus, M., Zinnikus, I., & Straube, S. (2016, September 12–13). Hybrid teams of humans, robots and virtual agents in a production setting. In *Proceedings of the 12th International Conference on Intelligent Environments, (IE-16), London.* IEEE.

Schwendner, J., Hidalgo, C. J., Domínguez, R., Planthaber, S., Yoo, Y. H., Asadi, B., Machowinski, J., Rauch, C., & Kirchner, F. (2015, May 11–13). Entern: Environment modelling and navigation for robotic space-exploration. In *Symposium on advanced space Technologies in Robotics and Automation (ASTRA), (ASTRA), Noordwijk, in proceedings ASTRA.*

Silver, D., Schrittwieser, J., Simonyan, K., Antonoglou, I., Huang, A., Guez, A., Hubert, T., Baker, L. R., Lai, M., Bolton, A., Chen, Y., Lillicrap, T. P., Hui, F. F., Sifre, L., Driessche, G. V., Graepel, T., & Hassabis, D. (2017). Mastering the game of Go without human knowledge. *Nature, 550,* 354–359.

Sonsalla, R., Cordes, F., Christensen, L., Roehr, T. M., Stark, T., Planthaber, S., Maurus, M., Mallwitz, M., & Kirchner, E. A. (2017, June 20–22). Field testing of a cooperative multi-robot sample return mission in Mars analogue environment. In *Proceedings of the 14th symposium on advanced space Technologies in Robotics and Automation (ASTRA 2017), (ASTRA-2017), Leiden, ESA.* ESA/ESTEC.

Yanco, H., & Drury, J. (2004). Classifying human-robot interaction: An updated taxonomy. In *Proceedings of the IEEE International Conference on Systems, Man and Cybernetics* (Vol. 3, pp. 2841–2846). Hague. https://doi.org/10.1109/ICSMC.2004.1400763

Sirko Straube studied neurobiology and computer science at the Albert-Ludwigs-University Freiburg, Germany, where he graduated in 2005. After completing his dissertation about human object recognition in 2009, he joined the Robotics Innovation Center in Bremen, Germany, first at the University Bremen—later at DFKI GmbH, leading projects focused on human–machine interaction, machine learning, hybrid teams of humans and robots, and advanced training for companies. Since 2015, Sirko Straube is the institute's deputy head. His core interests are in cooperation of industry and research, the successful knowledge transfer, and to bring more transparency about current AI-trends into the public awareness.

Nina Hoyer studied biology at the University of Oldenburg. In 2016, she completed her Dr.rer.nat in the field of neurobiology at the Center for Molecular Neurobiology, Hamburg (ZMNH). Since 2017, she started a position as a research associate at the Robotics Innovation Center at the German Research Center for Artificial Intelligence GmbH in Bremen, followed by research position at the Research Group Robotics of the University of Bremen. Her work focusses on the coordination and acquisition of projects.

Niels Will graduated as a physiotherapist and studied health sciences in Hamburg, Germany. Since 2011, he is as a research associate at the German Research Center for Artificial Intelligence GmbH in Bremen. His research focuses are on human–robot collaboration, e.g. robotic therapy and care systems or in terms of industrial and logistical applications. Until today, he leads various projects in the application areas and works in project coordination and acquisition.

Prof. Dr. Dr. h.c. Frank Kirchner is an Executive Director of the German Research Center for Artificial Intelligence, Bremen, and is responsible for the Robotics Innovation Center—one of the largest centers for AI and Robotics in Europe. Founded in 2006 as the DFKI Laboratory, it builds on the basic research of the Robotics Working Group headed by Kirchner at the University of Bremen. There, Kirchner holds the Chair of Robotics in the Department of Mathematics and Computer Science since 2002. Frank Kirchner is one of the leading experts in the field of biologically inspired behavior and motion sequences of highly redundant, multifunctional robot systems and machine learning for robotics control.

Open Access This chapter is licensed under the terms of the Creative Commons Attribution 4.0 International License (http://creativecommons.org/licenses/by/4.0/), which permits use, sharing, adaptation, distribution and reproduction in any medium or format, as long as you give appropriate credit to the original author(s) and the source, provide a link to the Creative Commons license and indicate if changes were made.

The images or other third party material in this chapter are included in the chapter's Creative Commons license, unless indicated otherwise in a credit line to the material. If material is not included in the chapter's Creative Commons license and your intended use is not permitted by statutory regulation or exceeds the permitted use, you will need to obtain permission directly from the copyright holder.

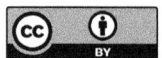

Chapter 5
The Legal Challenge of Robotic Assistance

Lorenz Kähler and Jörn Linderkamp

Abstract This chapter addresses the legal implications of robotic assistance. Artificial intelligence, which shall make decisions autonomously or act autonomously in interaction with humans, is associated with a substantial potential for conflict that will also and especially become evident from a legal point of view. The more AI diffuses into people's spheres of life, the more conflicts which are associated with it will become a major theme for both the legislator and the judiciary. Questions which they have to answer include who is liable in the case of an accident and how personal data recorded via robots might be used against the owner and for third parties, including government agencies. If robots carry out actions seemingly based on their own decisions the question arises whether robots are legal persons and acquire "personality" rights as a result. Building on the results from the Delphi expertise on the social conflict scenario, the chapter examines from a legal perspective the challenges that the diffusion of AI and robots brings with it in people's spheres of life.

Keywords Regulation of robots · Liability · Legal personhood · Right to human contact · Discrimination

5.1 Introduction

Every new technology raises new legal questions, the answers to which, however, will be similar in a surprising number of cases. This is also true where robots are concerned since a multitude of existing legal provisions, which have been developed and proven themselves over the centuries, can be applied to them. This is true, for example, for the contract of sale and the transfer of ownership. In all likelihood, in the future you must still pay a price for the purchase of a robot, ownership will also then typically only be transferred when the purchase price has been paid in full and

---

L. Kähler (✉) · J. Linderkamp
University of Bremen, Bremen, Germany
e-mail: lkaehler@uni-bremen.de

there will be warranty rights in the event of a defect. Similarly, the owner will continue to be entitled to handle a robot at his or her discretion, leave him unused or even destroy him, just as one is allowed to do with all other things owned.

Before we turn to the new legal questions raised by the use of robots, it makes sense to take a closer look at this phenomenon, i.e. that surprisingly often, new technology does not require new legal answers. For it is only against the background of this phenomenon that it becomes understandable at which points the use of robots entails new legal questions that cannot be dealt with by the existing norms. As the example of the contract of sale and the transfer of ownership demonstrate, the novelty of the technology alone is not sufficient to prove a need for legal reform.

The ability of existing law to regulate new technological developments is primarily due to its abstract character. The use of abstract terms makes it possible to regulate a wide range of previously unknown issues. Whether one buys a bread roll or a not yet existing quantum computer, decades-old wood or some newly developed material, is irrelevant for the norms of the contract of sale. In legal terms, all these are purchased objects, and robots should not be an exception since they are also objects, at least in accordance with the current legislation. Even if one were to argue that due to their ability to learn they might be compared to animals (e.g. Zech, 2020, p. 66), this would not change anything. For at least under German law, animals are also treated as material objects (cf. section 90a German Civil Code: BGB).

Due to general terms, the use of robots can often be regulated with the existing norms. This applies in particular with regard to contract and tort law. The latter is primarily based on the concept of negligence. Negligence is the central requirement for liability and is generally understood as a violation of the required due diligence, section 276 (2) BGB. What this due diligence consists of in detail depends on a variety of circumstances. These circumstances have not been prescribed by statutory law and may be subject to change, which leaves a wide scope of concretisation for the courts. Therefore, the courts already have the legal instruments to order liability for the use of robots whose technical characteristics are not yet known in detail.

For example, no new law is needed to deem it negligent if robots with unknown tactile abilities are used for the care of people without extensive prior tests. Given the serious risks for life and limb when robots are used in interaction with human beings, it would be also negligent not to install an emergency button or similar mechanism with which they could be quickly and easily switched off (cf. Söbbing, 2019, p. 148). While the technology and the accompanying risks may be new, their legal treatment is still based on the idea of not endangering anyone that has always been a core principle of law ("neminem laedere"). What these duties of due diligence consist of in detail is not decisive here. Rather, it is important to understand that not every new technological phenomenon requires new regulations since its legal assessment can remain unchanged in view of the consistency of the basic regulatory standards.

Nevertheless, new technologies often lead to the adoption of new regulations. The history of technology shows that the legislator rarely relies on the flexibility of existing standards. This was the case with the development of railways (in former Prussia, for example, the legislator enacted a statute as early as in 1838) as well as the spread of the Internet (for German law, e.g. the statute about tele-services in 1997).

In some constellations, such changes can indicate where existing law does not adequately cover the new technology. In part, however, such changes are simply due to the fact that the political public frequently underestimates the regulatory power of existing law and wrongly believes that a new phenomenon requires new norms and would otherwise remain unregulated.

Another reason why new norms are frequently provided for new technologies is their origin in political debate. Since such debate only works well if there is a pragmatic objective and the adoption of a law constitutes such an objective, political debate is often focussed on this. This leads to the creation of new laws with a regulatory content that goes hardly beyond existing law. Such legislative changes are less an expression of the need for regulation than of the wish of the political public to come to an understanding about these measures.

In order to discuss the legal challenges resulting from the use of robots, it is necessary to understand what is provided in this regard by existing law. Firstly, this includes an assessment of what existing abstract provisions mean for the use of robots. Secondly, it must be determined whether these provisions contain regulatory gaps which require new norms for the use of robots. Thirdly, it is worthwhile considering what the content of these new regulations should be in order to provide for the use of robots. While the first question is a legal one, the second and third question concern legal ethics. Therefore, they cannot be answered by an analysis of the applicable law alone, but require an answer to an ethical question that ultimately has to be decided politically, i.e. the question under which conditions robots may be used.

Since politics are in turn guided by the views of the population, one should make use of the findings of empirical social research when examining these questions. Surveys alone, of course, cannot determine the content of a future regulation. Rather, this requires legal and legal-ethical arguments, which can, however, build on the findings of empirical social research. The following legal discussion uses therefore the results of the 2019 Delphi presented in this book.

The following discussion will concentrate on the use of robots for consumers since the challenges in this field are particularly important. While the use of industrial robots has been common practice for some time, society has little experience so far with the use of robots in the domestic sector. Companies can be expected to have an expertise in dealing with robots, which cannot be readily assumed for consumers, especially if they need care. Consumers are not able to exchange, shut down, or reprogram robots. A further reason to focus on robots in the domestic sphere is that their use usually involves more personal and thus sensitive data than the use of robots in industry.

Among the issues raised by the use of robots for consumers, liability is of the greatest relevance. Frequently, there are concerns that with the increasing ability of robots to come to unforeseen decisions, human responsibility will end. Therefore, this issue is to be considered first (2.). Subsequently, it will be discussed whether robots can bear responsibility, too. This presupposes that they are treated as legal entities (3.). Regardless of how this question is answered, it has to be considered whether the data created by the use of robots are protected (4.). Further the question is raised whether there should be a right to be treated, at least to a minimum extent, by one's kind and thus by a natural person (5.). To conclude, it will be of use to consider what expectations there are for legal reforms (6.).

All these questions will be discussed against the background of German law. The legal situation in other European legal systems is likely to be similar as these are all historically in part based on Roman law and at present on EU law. But even if the answers provided by German law should diverge from those provided by other legal systems, they will demonstrate at least the issues that are raised by the use of robots.

In accordance with the ISO standard 8373:2012 2.6 a robot is referred to below as a machine performing movements through electronic control. Computers that merely process and output information, but do not perform movements, are therefore not treated as robots in the following. The same applies to electronic devices, such as refrigerators, telephones, or televisions, that are software-operated, but cannot move without human influence. This differentiation has the advantage that it avoids the difficult question of whether robots can act and decide independently. Even if one denies this, it may be observed that robots can perform movements without an immediate human input.

5.2 Liability

Progress in technology can easily be associated with an increase of risks, if only because the risks of new technologies are not known and thus feared more than familiar risks. Empirically, however, technical progress is generally more likely to lead to a reduction rather than an increase of risks. This is especially true for the use of robots in the domestic sector as this is not associated with the danger of incalculable damage, as in the case of construction of a dam or a nuclear power plant, since only one person or, in the worst case, a few people are affected. The risks associated with the use of robots are therefore only likely to occur from time to time while the associated gains in safety are a general outcome. Once a malfunction has occurred and been observed, robots of the same design can be turned off in order to prevent such damage in future cases.

All in all, the use of robots for consumers is therefore expected to lead to a reduction rather than an increase of risks. For example, a robot used in the care sector could indicate illnesses of a patient or the danger of a heart attack at an early stage and thus increase the safety of patients overall despite new risks. Nevertheless, the question of who is liable in the event of damage remains important. The overall reduction of risks cannot serve as an excuse for damage in the individual case.

Interestingly, the above-described association of new technology with an increase of risks has already resulted in the so-called strict liability being imposed for new technical devices in many other places. This liability differs from fault liability insofar as it does not depend on the culpable actions of individual persons. Such strict liability was provided early on for railways (section 1 Liability Act, HPflG), in later times for aircraft (sections 44, 45 Civil Aviation Act, LuftVG) and car accidents (section 7 Road Traffic Act, StVG). Strict liability also applies for drugs (section 84 Pharmaceutical Products Act, AMG). Such liability does not require proof that a specific person has violated his or her duty of care and is therefore to be blamed for something. In principle, it is sufficient that damage has been caused by the new technology.

On the one hand, this strict liability is based on the consideration that the person who significantly benefits from the use of new technology should also bear the associated risks (Deutsch, 1992, p. 74). On the other hand, those who are exposed to the new dangers related to the technology are to be protected. Moreover, incentives are to be set to invest into safety at an early stage. All this ultimately has the effect that people are significantly better protected against damages caused by technical products than against accidents caused by human error. Humans remain the greatest risk.

Of utmost relevance for the use of robots is the existing product liability, which is structured as strict liability (Deutsch, 1992, p. 73). Accordingly, liability arises if a defective product causes the death of a person, injury to the body or health of a person, or damage to an item of property, section 1 (1) Product Liability Act, ProdHaftG. A product is defective if it is constructed in such a way that its use can harm others. If damage is caused by a robot, the widespread hindsight bias (cf. Fischhoff, 1975, p. 288 ff) contributes to the assumption that different programming would have prevented the damage and that the robot is therefore defective. A technical failure is hardly ever classified as an unavoidable stroke of fate and thus acceptable. If, for example, a robot drops a person to be cared for, it will generally be assumed that the programming or the mechanics of that robot has been defective. It is not necessary to prove that a specific programmer or designer could have recognised this. Rather it is factually sufficient to show that a differently programmed or constructed robot would not have caused such damage.

Nevertheless, there is no product liability if a defect could not be detected at the time of sale in accordance with the state of scientific and technical knowledge, section 1 (2) no. 5 ProdHaftG. However, this is difficult to prove for the producer since technical expertise can usually show later on that the damage was caused by an error that could have been avoided. For completely new and unforeseen scientific phenomena are not the kind of events that occur in the use of new technology. This is particularly true for the use of robots since the risks associated with them are primarily related to the laws of mechanics and the employed program code. The laws of mechanics are well researched so that an error can hardly be traced by back to an inadequate knowledge at the time of sale. The same ultimately applies to a program code. It is a human creation which is not inevitable and could have been created differently. If any damage occurs during the use of robots, this is unlikely to be classified as unavoidable and accordingly, an exception to the otherwise applicable liability cannot be considered. At most, liability gaps could arise if the software of a third party, which is not liable as the producer, is installed on the robot after it has been put into operation. For such, as yet hypothetical cases, an extension of product liability would provide a solution (European Commission, 2020, p. 14).

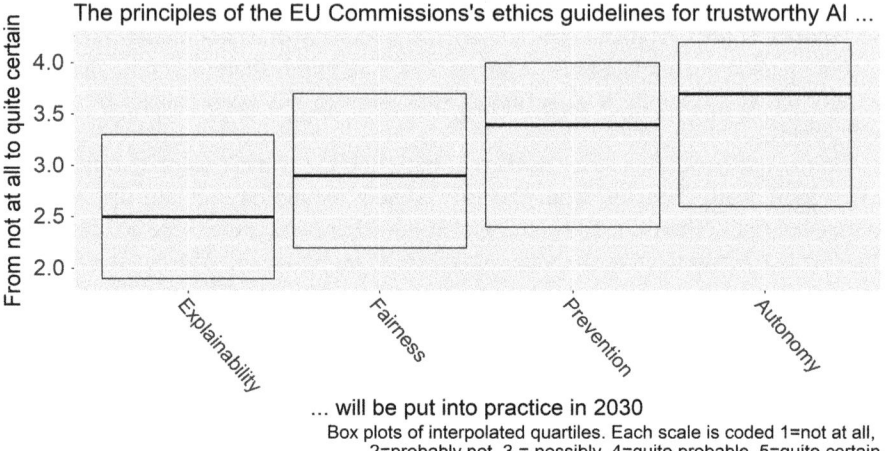

Fig. 5.1 Prediction about EU-Ethics guidelines for trustworthy AI

These considerations apply in particular to the use of robots in the domestic sector. Unlike robots used in industry, such robots regularly come into physical contact with human beings. This requires the use of the so-called soft robots, which are constructed to be more sensitive and submissive to human behaviour (Haddadin & Knobbe, 2020, p. 28). For care robots can cause damage through malfunction during physical contact, for example, through too intensive massaging or too much pressure on the patient. Since even a serious suspicion of dangers to life and limb entails a special duty of care (BGHZ 80, 186, 192), the producers of robots are exposed to considerable liability risks. This is all the more true since criminal liability may apply in parallel to civil liability for the damages that have occurred. A producer who places an unsafe robot on the market may end up paying not only for damages arising during its use but can also be punished for negligent physical injury or even negligent homicide. It is therefore to be expected that care robots are only brought on the market after extensive tests have been carried out and proved their use to be relatively safe.

Precautions against conceivable damages correspond to widely held expectations, as the Delphi has shown. Those questioned tended to rate it as possible up to "quite probable" that ethics guidelines of the European Commission call for damage prevention, i.e. that AI systems should neither cause nor aggravate damage (Fig. 5.1 and Table 5.1).

The duty to take precautions against damages is of the greatest relevance when it comes to the question of who is liable in the event of its violation. As a starting point, it is important to realise that these may be several different persons at the same time. The fact that the producer of a robot is liable for the damage caused by it does not exclude the liability of others. Contrary to a widespread view among laypersons, it is not necessary to decide whether either the producer or the programmer or the seller

Table 5.1 Predictions about EU-Ethics guidelines for trustworthy AI

Autonomy	The ethics guideline calls for autonomy: people must be able to retain full and effective self-determination about themselves. This principle could be put into practice.
Prevention	The ethics guideline calls for damage prevention: AI systems should neither cause nor aggravate damage. This principle could be put into practice.
Fairness	The ethics guideline calls for fairness: AI supports justice and protection against discrimination and stigmatisation. This principle could be put into practice.
Explainability	The ethics guideline calls for explainability: AI is transparent and can be explained. Its goals are communicated openly. This principle could be put into practice.

or even the robot is liable for the damage. As in many other cases of contractual or statutory liability, there may be a so-called joint and several liability, under which each injuring party is liable for the entire damage, section 426 BGB. This may, therefore, include all the persons mentioned above. Who bears which share is then determined in the internal relationship of the injuring parties. This is of little importance for the injured party, as he or she can choose who to claim damages from and to what extent.

If a robot causes damage to the health or property of a consumer, according to section 1 (1) Product Liability Act, at least the producer is liable for damages. This is based on Art. 1 of European Directive 85/374/EEC and therefore similar in all Member States of the EU. Liability arises irrespective of where the producer is located and whether he is the one who made the decision leading to the damage. Thus, even if the robot is seen to have caused the damage itself, the producer remains responsible as this does not call into question the fact that he or she manufactured the robot. It is not likely that this will change in the future although the development and dissemination of robots would be promoted if the liability of their producers was to be restricted. For the already mentioned conviction remains that producers profit from the sales of robots and that their use is associated with enormous risks.

The liability of the producer is complemented by the liability of the person under whose trademark the robot is distributed as he or she is also treated as the producer, section 4 (1) sentence 2 ProdHaftG. The person who is considered to be the producer in commercial transactions can therefore not exonerate himself or herself with the fact that the robot was manufactured by someone else. The same applies to a person who brings a robot onto the European market. Therefore, the responsibility cannot be delegated to a person from a non-European country where liability can hardly be enforced.

In addition to this producer's liability, there is fault-based tort liability, which can be based on all actions leading to damage and may therefore apply not only to the producer, but also the distributor and the seller as well as other persons or institutions involved in the usage of robots; for example, a care home. On the producer's side, mainly four types of errors lead to liability. Firstly, there are construction errors (BGH, NJW 1990, 906, 907), where liability arises if the planning of a robot has not sufficiently taken into account all risks. This would be, for example, the case if no emergency button or similar safety mechanism to switch off the robot had been provided. Planning would also be inadequate if a robot was unable to process the information that a human is standing in its way, and this would result in a collision.

Secondly, liability arises from manufacturing errors, which occur when a defect occurs in its production. This is especially the case if construction plans have been inadequately implemented, for example, because the defectiveness of the material was overlooked. Thirdly, liability arises where lacking or faulty instructions lead to damages (BGHZ 116, 60, 72–73).

Fourthly, inadequate product monitoring also leads to liability (BGHZ 99, 167, 171–172; NJW-RR 1995, 342, 343). This is based on the obligation to monitor whether any errors have occurred during the use of a product, especially if its technic is complex. In order to fulfil this obligation, producers can contact maintenance workshops, ascertain through purchaser surveys whether any problems have occurred, or follow reports in the press and on the Internet. This obligation to monitor products is only lowered if products have been on the market for a long time which is currently not the case for robots in the domestic sector.

As has been emphasised above, such a liability of the producer does not exclude the liability of the person who has sold or operates the robot. The seller and operators of the robot are therefore liable if, due to similar cases, they should have known that it can cause damages. In contrast, they are not liable under current law if damages suddenly occur and could not have been predicted by them. It has been proposed by some that the operator's liability should also be strict (Expert Group, 2019, p. 39). In addition, contractual liability may apply if a robot's use is based on a contract. This is, for example, the case in special-care homes. In general, this liability is also fault-based.

Irrespective of the type of liability, contributory negligence might decrease the amount of compensation. This is the case if a fault of the injured party has contributed to the occurrence of the damage, section 254 BGB. This is of particular importance for the liability of robots as their movements might also depend on how they are treated by their users. If a user instructs the robot to apply more pressure on her or his body, any damage occurring at a later stage might be caused by the robot having been taught this behaviour as normal. This does not place the responsibility on the user to teach the robot correct behaviour. However, it exempts the producer from liability for damages if it is apparent that these have been caused solely by incorrect use. Nevertheless, it should be noted that the producer of a product is also expected to take into account the possibility of incorrect use and can therefore not exonerate himself or herself with the fact that the user was warned against a certain use. In the example of pressure being applied on the body, an obvious precaution would be to limit the intensity of this pressure to a certain level regardless of the preferences of the user.

As these cases show liability depends on abstract concepts such as negligence and fault, which require concretisation with regard to the specific use of a robot. As has been observed above, this is a considerable advantage, on the one hand, since it allows for a flexible approach of the law to new technologies. On the other hand, it

Table 5.2 Delphi scenarios of ethical and legal challenges

Discrimination	Since AI made decisions about recruiting, discrimination, stigmatisation, and violation of personal rights when looking for a job have decreased significantly.
Creditworthiness	Since decisions have become AI-driven, the classification of creditworthiness not only include characteristics of the loan seeker himself; thus decisions on a loan have been increasingly challenged in courts in recent years.
Lifestyle	Since AI-supported lifestyle-related risk calculations have become the norm in the insurance industry, contract decisions by insurance companies have increasingly been challenged in court.
Liability	Clarification of liability issues in self-learning, autonomously acting AI systems is now up to the highest German court.
Permit	The EU ethics guideline has been a legal requirement for everyone to comply with since 2025. The AI assistance systems developed for recruitment of job seekers have since then to be officially approved to guarantee protection against discrimination, stigmatisation, and violation of personal rights.
Creature	Ethics committees are now seriously concerned with the question: "Is it still appropriate to legally view robots as a thing and not as a creature to be endowed with personal rights when they live in a common household with people?"
Deletion	Robots that specialise in communication in a person's home environment are now often rented rather than bought. The common practice of deleting all data that has accrued and learned from this environment, after termination of the tenancy, when the robot is rented out to the next customer has now met with serious ethical reservations.
Privacy	Requests from government agencies to be allowed to hack, without a justified reason, information from AI systems for surveillance and prevention purposes have always been rejected by the courts.

means that the drawing of specific boundaries will be left to the courts. Interestingly, this also corresponds to the expectations of those questioned in the Delphi, who considered it most likely among the various scenarios that in 2030 the "clarification of liability issues in self-learning, autonomously acting AI systems is now up to the highest German court" (Table 5.2).[1]

This expectation that liability will be clarified by the courts exceeds the expectation that "requests from government agencies to be allowed to hack, without a justified reason, information from AI systems for surveillance and prevention purposes have always been rejected by the courts". In addition to the expected need to clarify the legal details, this indicates an expectation that the use of robots is associated with a potential for damage and that questions of liability will therefore have to be resolved. It remains unclear, however, whether respondents were aware that this would primarily concern the details of liability and less the fundamental question of whether liability arises at all.

---

[1] We would like to thank Uwe Engel for the calculations and charts which are shown here.

Another interesting aspect of the respondents' expectations is their comparative uncertainty as to whether ethics committees in 2030 will be seriously concerned with the question: "Is it still appropriate to legally view robots as a thing and not as a creature to be endowed with personal rights when they live in a common household with people"? This uncertainty about the legal status of robots is well founded insofar as the latter is in general irrelevant for liability. Even if robots were treated as legal entities, as will be discussed below, this would not exclude the liability of the producer and the seller. Accordingly, it is not to be expected for future practice that liability for a robot will depend on its treatment as a legal person.

5.3 Legal Personhood

It would be a legal revolution if robots would be treated as separate legal entities. This question has therefore caused a wide debate (Solum, 1992, p. 1231 ff; Balkin, 2015, p. 55 ff; Ebers, 2020, p. 99). A starting point for it is the observation that, already today, robots are used for tasks which humans do not want to or are unable to perform (Balkin, 2015, p. 59). An example for this is software which detects melanoma more reliably than experienced physicians (Brinker et al., 2019, p. 47 ff). Robots seem thus to make decisions that were previously the responsibility of humans while acting in ways that humans find difficult to understand. Should they therefore legally be treated as persons?

Against this the objection suggests itself that robots are programmed and constructed by humans and, as artefacts, lack the ability to reproduce, which characterises living beings. However, this attribute is not decisive for the question of the legal personality of robots for two reasons. Firstly, it cannot be excluded, at least in theory, that robots in turn construct other robots (von Neumann, 1966, p. 79). Secondly, it is not evident why legal capacity should depend on the ability to reproduce. Independently upon this capacity humans have a legal status as persons because they are intrinsically valuable.

In addition to human beings, however, the law also treats other entities as legal persons, among them public limited companies and associations. None of these are natural persons as they lack essential human characteristics such as being able to act on their own. They always have to be represented by others. Nevertheless, they have rights and obligations and can therefore sue and be sued in courts. The fact that they are represented by human beings does not exclude their legal capacity any more than the legal capacity of an infant is called into question by the fact that it is represented by its parents in court.

Should robots therefore be represented by humans and treated as legal entities? Or would this call into question the dignity of human beings since the law would then grant robots the same rights? At least the respondents of the Delphi believe it to be probable that human self-determination will have to be protected in view of the advent of robots (Fig. 5.1). Interestingly, they are even more certain in this respect than as to whether ethical guidelines should be established in order to encourage damage prevention.

While human autonomy appears to be threatened in its exclusivity when there are other legal entities besides human beings, it may theoretically also be at risk if robots lack this quality. If they take over a multitude of decisions from humans and thus shape reality, it becomes important to defend oneself against their "actions" if those infringe one's liberty or property. Then legal personhood and thus the capacity of being sued could arguably help. However, this would only be necessary if, unlike under current law, there were no other responsible parties against whom a claim could be made (2).

Since robots differ from humans in central characteristics such as origin, sentience, and ability to develop, one might consider attributing legal personhood to them if they resembled legal persons. Such persons are characterised by the fact that they exist independently of their members or shareholders as well as objects belonging to them. In extreme cases, there may be legal entities such as the assetless association, which have no property and for which no people work. Legal persons are thus independent of their human founders and the material objects belonging to them. Such independence does not exist in the case of robots. They are programmed by humans and equipped with hardware. Accordingly, they remain objects that depend upon their material substance, although they exist independently of their developers and operators to some extent (Borges, 2018, p. 978).

The dependency upon its material substance is particularly obvious in the fact that the existence of a robot can be terminated at any time by its destruction. This is different in the case of a legal person, which comes into being and ceases to exist only by a decision of the legal system. If the material objects belonging to a legal person are destroyed, this legal person does not cease to exist.

According to current law robots lack the ability to have rights and obligations, as do all other material objects and every animal, irrespective of any other properties they may possess. Therefore, even if robots had completely different technical properties, such as the ability to develop further and the ability to reproduce, they would not automatically be legal persons. The decisive question is therefore not a legal, but a legal-ethical one, namely whether robots should have their own rights and obligations. Technically, this is possible, just as some legal systems have already granted rights to animals and rivers, e.g. to the river Río Atrato at the transition to the Central American landmass (Talbot-Jones, 2021, p. 208). The question therefore is whether there are good reasons for recognising the legal capacity of robots. In the case of human beings, legal capacity is ultimately based on their intrinsic value, i.e. they deserve protection for their own sake. This does not apply in the case of robots, regardless of their level of technical development. Among other things, this is because they lack consciousness and are therefore unable to set themselves a purpose and experience the world in a conscious way. Rather, they are subject to the programmer's specifications, for example, in the question of what is to be learned (Zech, 2020, p. 42).

Being guided by human objectives, robots act for the benefit of a third party. It is not conceivable how this benefit of a third party could be promoted by robots being

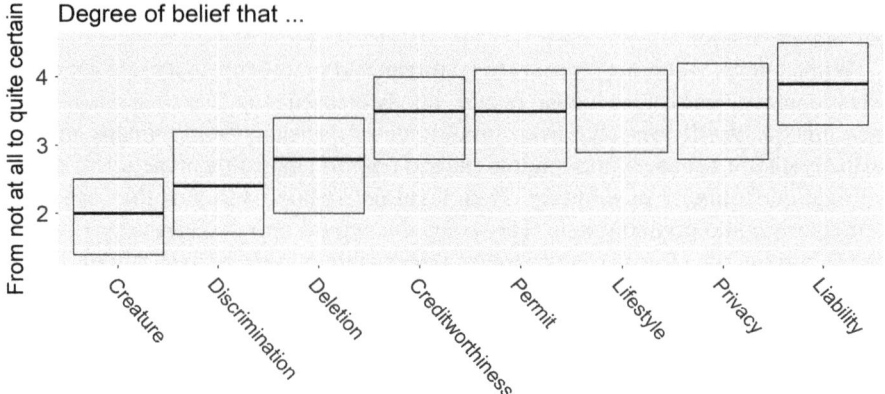

Fig. 5.2 Delphi scenarios of ethical and legal challenges

granted their own legal personality. Rather, it appears that the best approach to ensure this is to treat robots as objects that their owners may dispose of at will, section 903 BGB. People benefit from this either directly, if they own the robot, or indirectly, if they are a member or shareholder of a legal entity that owns the robot. This ensures that the legal system ultimately only promotes human interests. Denying legal capacity to robots ensures that this remains so. The state of technical development is not important in this context, since the ultimate reason for legal capacity is not a specific technical capability, but the promotion of human interest. The discussion on how the law should treat robots is therefore focused on liability, not on possible robot rights. Interestingly, this corresponds to the expectations of the Delphi respondents who do not tend to anticipate that ethics committee will be concerned with the question of whether a robot is a "creature to be endowed with personal rights" (Fig. 5.2).

The question of whether robots should be able to appear in court as plaintiffs also shows that it is not their technical capability which matters here. For it is not relevant whether they would be able to formulate and substantiate a legal claim, which seems at least conceivable with the appropriate development of software. Rather, the question is whether this would promote human interests. This is the case when human beings themselves act as plaintiffs and formulate their claims. The same applies if a legal person acts as plaintiff as it represents human beings or furthers their interest by enforcing its rights. Therefore, recognising the ability of legal persons to act as plaintiffs in court ultimately promotes human interests while it is not evident that the recognition of a corresponding capacity of robots could promote human interests at all.

These difficulties associated with treating robots as legal persons have led the European Parliament (European Parliament, 2017, no. 59–60) and some authors to argue that they should be granted partial legal capacity (Teubner, 2018, p. 204 f;

Schirmer, 2016, p. 663; Specht & Herold, 2018, p. 43). This would include the positive allocation of the rights and obligations required to deal with the digital entity in legal transactions and exclude others. For example, robots could be liable, but would not be able to form a limited company. Other authors have rejected this proposal (Expert Group, 2019, p. 38; Riehm, 2020, p. 47; Linke, 2021, p. 203; cf. www.robotics-openletter.eu), and with good reason, since the "actions" of robots can always be attributed to the producer or the operator. Therefore, there is a comprehensive liability regime (2.). Due to strict product liability and the parallel responsibility of different actors, it is not likely that there will be gaps in liability with regard to the use of robots. For instance, if a care robot injures a patient during treatment, the patient would therefore be sufficiently protected.

However, other authors assume a "responsibility gap" between the action of robots and civil liability (Teubner, 2018, p. 157 ff). This is said to arise because robots are supposedly able to act on their own authority and cause damage to the rights or legal interests of others. In this perspective, the human being in the background could not be accused of breaching a duty of care. Therefore, robots themselves would have to be held responsible. As the argument goes, the recognition of a partial legal capacity would avoid the unilateral passing-on of risks to the injured party.

However, firstly, this argument fails to recognise that fault does not only occur where an action directly leads to damage. Once a robot is deployed, it may no longer be possible for the designer or the seller to control its movements. In the case of self-learning systems, it may indeed be unpredictable how they behave. Liability, however, may already arise from the decision to use such an unpredictable machine. It would be negligent not to provide safety precautions such as a switch-off button or a corresponding code word ("Siri, stop!") to prevent damage. Secondly, product liability does not depend on fault in any case and a liability gap is therefore not plausible.

Also, it is inconceivable how a robot could have recoverable assets. If a robot causes significant damage, it is questionable whether it can still be used and has a monetary value because hardly anyone would be prepared to pay for its acquisition. Similarly, even a recognition of partial legal capacity does not ensure that robots have sufficient property. The insolvency risk in the event of damage is therefore enormous (Ebers, 2020, p. 102). If robots had significant assets and did not belong to any particular person, others would be allowed to appropriate them, section 958 (1) BGB. This could only be prevented if robots were recognised as something that deserves protection for its own sake. However, as shown above, there is no reason for this.

In German private law, the concept of partial legal capacity is not altogether unknown, but nevertheless an alien element. A frequently cited example is the unborn human being (nasciturus) who can inherit and thus establish own rights (section 1923 (2) BGB; Mayinger, 2017, pp. 179 f). However, the recognition of the capacity to inherit only serves to bridge the time between conception and birth and is aimed at the human to be born, not at the nasciturus' own interests. The nasciturus's capacity to inherit is not related to any significant liability either. The representatives of the nasciturus may disclaim the inheritance and thus release her or him from inherited debts (sections 1942 ff BGB) so that there is little risk of a financial burden. An analogy to the nasciturus is therefore not helpful with regard to the use of robots which are supposed to have duties.

If the objective of partial legal capacity is not the additional liability of robots, but an exemption from the liability of the owner, a liability privilege for the owner or operator would be sufficient. A new legal construct of partial legal capacity of robots is not required in this regard. Such a privilege would more clearly express the purpose of relieving owners. However, this effect shows the doubtful nature of such a privilege, since it is hardly understandable why the owners or operators of a robot should be exempted from the risks associated with its use while retaining the profits resulting from it. It is implausible why uninvolved third parties should bear the risks arising from an accidental meeting with a robot.

To conclude, the legal personhood of robots may inspire the imagination and generate new legal ideas. However, it cannot fix a problem of the current law. In this respect, the discussion of legal personhood for robots resembles science fiction literature, which is also inspiring, but not a reliable source for information about physics, technology, or law.

5.4 Data Protection

The handling of the personal data that is continuously collected by robots also raises pressing legal questions. Care robots, for example, analyse the environment via cameras and sensors, and register the intentions of the persons cared for (Steinrötter, 2020, p. 336). Such robots store detailed data about those requiring care; for example, data on their state of health or personal secrets entrusted to them. This includes first of all health data: who takes which medication, in what dose and how frequently? Who has undiagnosed high blood pressure? In addition to this, robots communicate with those in need of care. They can already perform simple communication tasks today, for example, via integrated speech recognition software (Steinrötter, 2020, p. 336).

Due to the extent and the sensitivity of the collected data, two fundamental rights are legally relevant, which have been developed over time by the Constitutional Court: the right to informational self-determination (BVerfGE 65, 1, 43) and the fundamental right to the confidentiality and integrity of information technology systems (BVerfG, NJW 2008, 822, 824). The former is of particular relevance for the processing of data. It is regulated by the binding provisions of the General Data Protection Regulation (GDPR) and is in turn flanked by the right to privacy of Art. 7 para. 1 of the Charter of Human Rights of the European Union and Art. 8 para. 1 of the European Convention on Human Rights.

The central question with regard to data protection in the use of robots is to whom the data processing can be attributed. If this is the data subject herself or himself, there are no restrictions set by data protection law. A robot that one has purchased or rented for one's personal use and the actions of which one can determine, can therefore also collect sensitive health data, for example, by measuring blood pressure or by taking photos.

However, this is not the case if the data processing is attributed to other persons, in particular if a care home, operates the robot and reads out and processes its data. In such cases, the data processing always requires justification, which may be provided by consent, Art. 6 lit. a) GDPR. If health data are concerned, consent must be expressed or data processing must be necessary for the provision of medical care, Art. 9 para. 2 lit. a), h) GDPR. The capacity to give consent is problematic, for example, when patients suffering from dementia or severe psychosis are concerned. In this case, consent can be provided by a guardian, or a living will made in advance (Steinrötter, 2020, p. 339).

If no effective consent of the data subject or his or her guardian can be established, processing may nevertheless be permitted. Firstly, this applies if the processing is a prerequisite for treatment in healthcare, Art. 9 para. 2 lit. h) GDPR. Secondly, data has to be stored in order to fulfil the obligation of documentation under tort law, which also serves to avert future damage.

Provided that no health data are concerned, data processing is also permitted according to Art. 6 lit. b) GDPR if required for the fulfilment of a contract. A robot is therefore permitted to record and process all data that promote the purposes of a contract, such as enabling communication, which opens up wide possibilities for data processing. Consequently, only a few cases are conceivable in which handling the collected data would clearly not be necessary according to the purpose of the contract. For example, the operator of a care robot would not be permitted to use the robot to collect data on any criminal offences committed by the patient if these were unrelated to the objective of communication.

In view of this variety of options to enable data processing, it is important to protect the collected data from external access by third parties who at first glance have nothing to do with the use of the robots. This applies in particular for the state accessing data for security reasons and for purposes of criminal prosecution.

The legal situation can be illustrated with the example of a person in need of care confessing the murder of his wife to a robot. Can the police and the department of public prosecution access the data if the offender was in full possession of his mental powers when confessing? In their collection of evidence, they have to make an important distinction, which is already laid down in the decisions of the Constitutional Court on a diary (BVerfGE 80, 367 ff) and of the Federal Court of Justice on self-talk (BGHSt 57, 71 ff). In both cases, the suspect had disclosed details of a crime committed by him. In the self-talk case, the suspect was sitting on his own in the car while being monitored by the law-enforcing authorities by means of technical devices without his knowledge on the basis of section 100f German Code of Criminal Procedure, StPO. He spoke to himself uttering compromising words, which later identified him as the perpetrator in the charged murder case.

In the diary case, the accused was suspected of beating a woman to death. He had hidden records, similar to a diary, in the house of his parents. These included indications of his problematic relationship with women, which the court regarded as incriminating evidence. While the Constitutional Court judged the diary to be admissible evidence (BVerfGE 80, 367, 376), the Federal Court of Justice rejected this in the self-talk case by assuming an independent prohibition of such a use of evidence (BGHSt 57, 71, 74).

The difference cannot consist in the disclosure of private information as such. Secrets may also be found in a diary. The author of a diary generally does not want others to read his or her intimate thoughts. Rather the decisive factor is the circumstance of feeling unobserved. The driver of a car without passengers may generally trust that no one is listening to him. The human dignity, as guaranteed by Art. 1 Basic Law, protects this personal space from the law enforcement authorities, even though this may impede the investigation of criminal offences (BGHSt 57, 71, 75). The author of the diary, in contrast, has to expect that someone might get hold of the written record (cf. BVerfGE 80, 367, 376), even if it is on the occasion of a house search. Unlike the spoken word, the written word is not transient.

This distinction can be used for the collection of robot data for purposes of criminal prosecution: If the person concerned had to expect the collection of her or his personal data, there is no general prohibition of data processing since the most personal sphere of life then is not affected. However, if the person concerned did not have to expect that his or her data of his most personal sphere would be collected, the constellation is similar to that of self-talk, the recording of which may not be used.

The robot might possibly be a welcome interlocutor. But the user should not in vain assume that her or his spoken word will remain transient and not be recorded for posterity. As far as the most personal sphere is concerned, section 100d (1) StPO explicitly requires that the personal data will not be used by the law enforcement authorities. If an attempt to deceive is involved because the care robot is falsely labelled as defective, for example, the collection of evidence is prohibited according to section 136a (3) StPO.

However, for data outside the most private sphere a robot may be accessed without the knowledge of its user, if he or she is suspected of a particularly serious crime (e.g. murder, aggravated robbery) and the course of events or the whereabouts of the accused cannot be established otherwise or only with great difficulty, section 100b StPO. These provisions show that the accessing of robot data is subject to considerable, though not insurmountable legal restrictions.

The law thus provides some protection against access to a robot's records, as this requires at least a justification by law or explicit consent. Against this background, the participants of the Delphi are surprisingly certain that an intervention in artificial intelligence systems will not take place without such a justification (Fig. 5.2). Whether this expectation is confirmed will not only depend on the applicable law, but also on its consistent implementation.

5.5 Right to Human Contact

People react to robots with a certain sympathy and affection if they are designed to be humanoid. This might result in a reality that is a horror scenario for the vast majority of people: a care home where a multitude of robots move around, but not a single human being, except for the people to be cared for. In such cases, those in need of care would be even more likely to treat robots as persons because of the lack of human contacts.

Such a scenario of "being alone among robots" raises the question of whether this may be compatible with the guarantee of human dignity provided by Art. 1 para. 1 GG. Because of their social nature, human beings should not be forced to spend their existence in total isolation (Stöger, 2020, p. 136 f). They rely on communication with their fellow human beings (European Parliament, 2017, no. 32). These requirements do not only prohibit the state to isolate people. Rather, the state must also actively protect human dignity, Art. 1 para. 1 sentence 2 GG. This includes actions to prevent such a situation in which people are only surrounded by robots. Insofar, there is right to a minimum of human contact.

This right prevents an unrestricted technicalisation of care. In particular people in need of care who, due to their lack of mobility, can hardly get into contact with others, have to be treated in a way that allows for a minimum of human contact. Robots cannot altogether replace human carers (Deutscher Ethikrat, 2020, p. 51) since they lack the empathy to put themselves in the situation of a person requiring care. Nevertheless, they can provide an important service in the care sector.

The right to a minimum of human contact does not exclude the use of robots in many areas of care and for other domestic tasks, if only because an essential aspect of care and domestic work consists in addressing hygienic and physical, but not communicative needs. A cleaner is not primarily expected to be entertaining or communicating. Accordingly, there is no constitutional guarantee that all domestic or care work will be undertaken by human beings and that there will be extensive human contact. It is primarily a question of political and private decisions how services are provided. Therefore, it depends very much on the resources that private individuals and the society are prepared to use for care. Only very few requirements are provided by the constitution in this respect.

5.6 Challenges for Law and Ethics

If one considers the various legal and ethical challenges once again, it becomes apparent that the use of robots in the domestic and the care sector is already regulated by a large number of provisions. At least with regard to the fundamental decisions of the legal system for extensive strict liability in the use of technology, the rejection of legal personhood for robots, and the protection of personal data in their use, a fundamental legal reform does not seem to be necessary. This does not exclude

Table 5.3 Principal component analysis of the ratings in Fig. 5.2

	PC1	PC2	PC3	PC4
	Standardised factor loadings			
Discrimination	0.03	0.06	0.02	0.93
Creditworthiness	0.85	−0.16	−0.01	−0.02
Lifestyle	0.83	0.17	0.00	0.05
Liability	0.18	0.27	0.42	−0.33
Permit	−0.08	0.08	0.78	−0.09
Creature	−0.17	0.83	−0.02	0.13
Deletion	0.17	0.81	−0.03	−0.04
Privacy	0.04	−0.20	0.73	0.18

Principal Component Analysis, $N = 118$; oblique rotation 4 (nearly uncorrelated) factors with Eigenvalue ≥ 1.0 extracted. Explained variance: 68%

revisions of some details, such as those currently discussed at the suggestion of the European Commission (European Commission, 2020). This includes, in particular, an explicit liability of robot operators (Zech, 2020, pp. 81, 101) and the introduction of a compulsory insurance system (European Parliament, 2017, no. 57–59). Such changes can be initiated by the legislator. In many cases, however, it will be left to the courts to clarify the details, as in other areas, by defining concrete requirements such as liability for negligence or defective products on the basis of the abstract provisions.

This concretisation by the courts corresponds to the expectations of the Delphi respondents insofar as they expect court proceedings with considerable certainty both for the decision on a person's creditworthiness when applying for a loan and for the calculation of the risks associated with a person's lifestyle by the insurance industry (Fig. 5.2). As a "principal component analysis" shows the answers to both questions can be traced back to a considerable extent to a common factor (PC1) (Table 5.3):

It seems fair to assume that the PC1 factor expresses the willingness to have legal issues clarified in court if significant economic consequences depend on this. This is firstly the case with decisions on creditworthiness since the credit instalments to be paid by a borrower depend on the standards applied. Therefore, if the courts prohibit the consideration of certain circumstances—such as a conviction that has already been erased from the criminal record—this can have a significant economic impact on the borrower.

Secondly, the same applies for the expectation examined in the Delphi as to whether the processing of data on the lifestyle of the insured party will be subject to legal proceedings in the future. This also has considerable economic consequences, namely the amount of insurance premiums to be paid. Accordingly, it may be worthwhile to have the courts review what data insurance companies are allowed to use. It is conceivable, for example, that courts may prohibit insurance companies from negatively considering the policyholder's contact with convicted criminals in his or her own family when calculating insurance premiums as it would make the rehabilitation of criminal offenders more difficult if even their own relatives were to avoid them. It is therefore not surprising that this question regarding the assessment of recreational behaviour is judged similarly to that of a person's creditworthiness. Both questions involve issues of economic significance, which cannot be clarified by the legislator but only by the courts.

Another interesting coincidence in the respondents' answers becomes visible when two further questions are assessed. The first is whether ethics committees will in future be confronted with the question of whether robots are still treated as objects and not as creatures endowed with personal rights. The second question is whether the deletion of data on termination of a robot lease, which has so far been common practice, will meet with ethical concerns in the future. Both scenarios are characterised by a deviation from ethical principles that have been considered mostly plausible up to now. In the first case, this is the treatment of robots as objects, in the second, the systematic processing of personal data.

The apparent scepticism towards these scenarios might therefore be based in both cases on the assumption that ethical principles, unlike technology, hardly change. This assumption could be indicated by a principal component PC2. If one considers the topicality of debates on justice, which have been led since ancient times, the assumption appears justified. As much as robots revolutionise technology and require the adaptation of the details of legal provisions, they are not likely to change legal and ethical principles.

Appendix

Table 5.4 The quartiles graphed in Fig. 5.1

First Quartile	Second Quartile (median)	Third Quartile	
2.6	3.7	4.2	Autonomy
2.4	3.4	4	Prevention
2.2	2.9	3.7	Fairness
1.9	2.5	3.3	Explainability

Table 5.5 The quartiles graphed in Fig. 5.2

First Quartile	Second Quartile (median)	Third Quartile	
1.7	2.4	3.2	Discrimination
2.8	3.5	4	Creditworthiness
2.9	3.6	4.1	Lifestyle
3.3	3.9	4.5	Liability
2.7	3.5	4.1	Permit
1.4	2	2.5	Creature
2	2.8	3.4	Deletion
2.8	3.6	4.2	Privacy

References

Balkin, J. B. (2015). The path of robotics law. *California Law Review Circuit, 6*(June), 45–60.
Borges, G. (2018). Rechtliche Rahmenbedingungen für autonome Systeme. *Neue Juristische Wochenschrift, 71*(14), 978–982.
Brinker, T. J., et al. (2019). Deep learning outperformed 136 of 157 dermatologists in a head-to-head dermoscopic melanoma image classification task. *European Journal of Cancer, 113*(May), 47–54.
Deutsch, E. (1992). Das neue System der Gefährdungshaftungen: Gefährdungshaftung, erweiterte Gefährdungshaftung und Kausal-Vermutungshaftung. *Neue Juristische Wochenschrift, 45*(2), 73–77.
Deutscher Ethikrat. (2020, March 10). *Robotik für gute Pflege*. Stellungnahme. Retrieved January 18, 2022, from https://www.ethikrat.org/fileadmin/Publikationen/Stellungnahmen/deutsch/stellungnahme-robotik-fuer-gute-pflege.pdf
Ebers, M. (2020). Regulierung von KI und Robotik. In M. Ebers, C. Heinze, T. Krügel, & B. Steinrötter (Eds.), *Künstliche Intelligenz und Robotik* (1st ed., pp. 82–140). C.H. Beck.
European Commission. (2020). *Report on the safety and liability implications of Artificial Intelligence, the Internet of Things and robotics, COM(2020) 64 final*.
European Parliament. (2017). *Civil law rules on robotics, P8_TA(2017)0051*.
Expert Group on Liability and New Technologies – New Technologies Formation. (2019). *Liability for Artificial Intelligence and other emerging technologies*. Academic Press. https://doi.org/10.2838/573689
Fischhoff, B. (1975). Hindsight ≠ foresight: The effect of outcome knowledge on judgment under uncertainty. *Journal of Experimental Psychology: Human Perception and Performance, 1*(3), 288–299.
Haddadin, S., & Knobbe, D. (2020). Grundlagen und Anwendungen der Robotik. In M. Ebers, C. Heinze, T. Krügel, & B. Steinrötter (Eds.), *Künstliche Intelligenz und Robotik* (1st ed., pp. 1–37). C.H. Beck.
Linke, C. (2021). Die elektronische Person. Erforderlichkeit einer Rechtspersönlichkeit für autonome Systeme? *Multimedia und Recht, 24*(3), 200–204.
Mayinger, S. M. (2017). *Die künstliche Person*. Fachmedien Recht und Wirtschaft.
Riehm, T. (2020). Nein zur ePerson! Gegen die Anerkennung einer digitalen Rechtspersönlichkeit. *Recht Digital, 1*(1), 42–47.
Schirmer, J. (2016). Rechtsfähige Roboter? *Juristenzeitung, 71*(13), 660–666.
Söbbing, T. (2019). *Fundamentale Rechtsfragen zur künstlichen Intelligenz (AI Law)*. Fachmedien Recht und Wirtschaft.
Solum, L. B. (1992). Legal personhood for artificial intelligences. *North Carolina Law Review, 70*(4), 1231–1287.
Specht, L., & Herold, S. (2018). Roboter als Vertragspartner? Gedanken zu Vertragsabschlüssen unter Einbeziehung automatisiert und autonom agierender Systeme. *Multimedia und Recht, 21*(1), 40–44.
Steinrötter, B. (2020). Datenschutzrechtliche Implikationen beim Einsatz von Pflegerobotern. Frühzeitig eingeholte Einwilligungen als Schlüssel für zulässige Geriatronik-Anwendungen. *Zeitschrift für Datenschutz, 10*(7), 336–340.
Stöger, K. (2020). Dürfen Maschinen menschliche Barmherzigkeit ersetzen? *LIMINA – Grazer Theologische Perspektiven, 3*(2), 131–148. Retrieved January 18, 2022, from https://limina-graz.eu/index.php/limina/article/view/76

Talbot-Jones, J. (2021). Advancing water law through rights of nature. In J. W. Dellapenna & J. Gupta (Eds.), *Water law* (1st ed., pp. 203–213). Edward Elgar.

Teubner, G. (2018). Digitale Rechtssubjekte? Zum privatrechtlichen Status autonomer Softwareagenten. *Archiv für die civilistische Praxis, 218*(2–4), 155–205.

von Neumann, J. (1966). *Theory of self-reproducing automata*. University of Illinois Press.

Zech, H. (2020). *Entscheidungen digitaler autonomer Systeme: Empfehlen sich Regelungen zu Verantwortung und Haftung? Gutachten A zum 73. Deutschen Juristentag*. C.H. Beck.

Lorenz Kähler, born in 1973, studied law and philosophy in Heidelberg, London, and Göttingen. Ph.D. in law about overruling decisions in 2003; habilitation about the justification and concept of default rules in 2010, Ph.D. in philosophy about duties to oneself in 2021. Since 2011, Professor for Private Law, Civil Procedure, and Legal Philosophy at the University of Bremen. Main research area: contract theory and the social ontology of law.

Jörn Linderkamp, born in 1989, studied law in Osnabrück (Germany) and Ljubljana (Slovenia). After practical experience as a judge, he has been a doctoral candidate at the University of Bremen since 2018. There he researches and publishes on topics of digital law. His doctoral thesis deals with personalised pricing and the opportunities and limits of artificial intelligence.

Open Access This chapter is licensed under the terms of the Creative Commons Attribution 4.0 International License (http://creativecommons.org/licenses/by/4.0/), which permits use, sharing, adaptation, distribution and reproduction in any medium or format, as long as you give appropriate credit to the original author(s) and the source, provide a link to the Creative Commons license and indicate if changes were made.

The images or other third party material in this chapter are included in the chapter's Creative Commons license, unless indicated otherwise in a credit line to the material. If material is not included in the chapter's Creative Commons license and your intended use is not permitted by statutory regulation or exceeds the permitted use, you will need to obtain permission directly from the copyright holder.

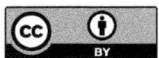

Chapter 6
Cognition-Enabled Robots Assist in Care and Everyday Life: Perspectives, Challenges, and Current Views and Insights

Michael Beetz, Uwe Engel, and Hagen Langer

Abstract The chapter focuses on research on robotic assistants and the involved challenge of their manipulating the physical world. It describes the state of the art in this regard and outlines directions for future research. Furthermore, it reports how the Delphi respondents assess various facets of human–robot communication and how specifically the group of scientists from engineering and natural sciences assesses the further technical development of 13 robotic skills. For this aspect, we asked for the experts' assessment of the points in time when robots will presumably be capable of demonstrating such skills. The list of examples includes cognitive and communicative skills and skills that relate to motion, autonomous navigation, and the performance of everyday activities at home/in elderly care. In addition, the chapter reports on findings from the population survey. It particularly reveals the relative importance that people allocate to the skills of care robots. It underlines the importance of considering the impact of the physical design of a robot on its social perception and acceptance.

Keywords Everyday Activity Science and Engineering · EASE Robot Household Marathon Experiment · Hybrid knowledge representation and reasoning · Cognition-enabled robots · Communication with robots · Robotic skills: By when · Expected skills of care robots

6.1 Robotic Assistants: Challenges, State of the Art, and Future Research

The design and realization of robotic agents that can master everyday activities, such as setting a table for breakfast, loading a dishwasher, and preparing a simple meal at human level, is still a very challenging task. Despite many recent advances in Artificial Intelligence, there are many yet unsolved problems. In this section, we

---

M. Beetz · U. Engel (✉) · H. Langer
University of Bremen, Bremen, Germany
e-mail: uengel@uni-bremen.de

© The Author(s) 2023
U. Engel (ed.), *Robots in Care and Everyday Life*, SpringerBriefs in Sociology,
https://doi.org/10.1007/978-3-031-11447-2_6

will examine why the development of autonomous general-purpose robot agents is such a complex and challenging task. We will also briefly sketch the current state of the art of the field, and how future research in AI and robotics could address these problems and overcome the existing barriers through the development of novel cognitive architectures and integrated hybrid knowledge bases for robots, which combine symbolic knowledge, fine-grained physical simulation of the real world, and powerful reasoning methods.

6.1.1 The Challenge of Manipulating the Physical World

The need to change the physical world to achieve one's goals is arguably one of the key driving forces behind the cognitive development of the human brain (Wolpert, 2011). Therefore, creating robot agents with human-level competence in goal-directed manipulation of objects and substances has been, is, and will continue to be one of the grand research challenges in AI and robotics (Kuipers et al., 2017). We can appreciate the magnitude of this challenge by looking at the breadth and depth of skill with which humans accomplish tasks, such as pouring substances: humans can pour water out of a pot and pancake mix into a pan; they can separate egg yolk from the egg white, extinguish fire, neutralize acid, and pour beer into a glass, to name only a few variations. These pouring tasks involve different substances being poured, different containers, and different tools. They serve different purposes and have different effects. Each variation of the pouring task requires its own specific behavior patterns.

Everyday manipulation tasks are usually stated in general vague terms. For example, when you are asked to "extinguish the fire" you have to translate this underdetermined task request into a context-specific body motion (to pour water on the fire) that is expected to achieve the desired effects and minimize the risks of unwanted side effects. This contextualization of underdetermined tasks is one of the most fundamental and challenging cognitive tasks that the human brain is capable of. The human brain harnesses powerful prospection capabilities (Williams, 2018; Szpunar et al., 2014; Jeannerod, 2001) to ensure that this contextualization typically succeeds on the first attempt, even for novel objects, tools, and context conditions and complex tasks. A number of researchers have stressed the essential role of prospection for effective agency. For example, Craik (1943) stated "If the organism carries a 'small-scale model' of external reality and of its own possible actions within its head, it is able to try out various alternatives, conclude which is the best of them, react to future situations before they arise, utilise the knowledge of past events in dealing with the present and future, and in every way to react in a much fuller, safer, and more competent manner to the emergencies which face it."

The power of prospection becomes particularly evident in open-ended manipulation task learning when humans learn manipulation tasks that require flexible, robust, and context-sensitive behavior in very few and often even in a single attempt by watching task demonstrations (Laird et al., 2017). Humans can learn manipulation tasks so efficiently because they can understand why the demonstrated behavior achieves the task, they have intuitions about the physical properties of objects to be acted on and expectations of their physical behavior when manipulated, they can imagine how they would generate the behavior for a demonstrated action, they anticipate the effects of the envisioned behavior even for hypothetical conditions, they transfer the observed behavior to their own bodies, objects, tasks, and contexts, and they adapt specific sub-motions to ensure task success.

While researchers across many disciplines appreciate the key role of prospection for effective agency (Szpunar et al., 2014; Vernon, 2014; Jeannerod, 2001; McDermott, 1992; Nau et al., 2004; Shanahan, 2006), the design and realization of computational models—knowledge representation and reasoning (KR&R) frameworks—that can exhibit the prospection capabilities that suffice for the one-shot contextualization of underdetermined manipulation tasks is an uncharted, high-gain research challenge.

6.1.2 State of the Art

Software agents have learned world champion level skills in playing Go (Silver et al., 2016; Schrittwieser et al., 2019), even with minimal hand-coded knowledge (Silver et al., 2017) or when learning other (Mnih et al., 2015; Schrittwieser et al., 2019) including Dota2, a multi-player video game that requires complex, continuous actions (Berner et al., 2019). The learning of physical actions was tackled; for example, tasks such as solving Rubik's cube (OpenAI, 2019) and picking up objects (Levine et al., 2018). These breakthroughs were obtained by combining novel deep artificial neural network (reinforcement) learning architectures, methods for generating huge amounts of training data or playing training games, and the computing power needed to learn complex tasks based on these data. These impressive performance breakthroughs do not mean that these technologies on their own can scale up to open-ended manipulation task learning (Marcus & Davis, 2021; Marcus, 2020). Perhaps the most obvious reason is that any manipulation task learning method has to avoid manipulation failures during learning as much as possible, but failure is an intrinsic part of deep reinforcement learning.

Learning as model building and improvement has recently gained momentum in the context of investigating computational models of cognitive development from babies to toddlers (Lake et al., 2016). Here, some models suggest that the learning agent starts with core knowledge about objects, actions, numbers, and space (Spelke & Kinzler, 2009; Spelke, 2000) and a "game engine in the brain" (Ullman et al., 2017; Schwettmann et al., 2018) as its native knowledge sources and apply learning strategies inspired by the metaphors of the "child as a scientist" (Ullman & Tenenbaum, 2020) and "child as a hacker" (Rule et al., 2020). This research direction proposes machine learning methods with much higher training data efficiency, better transferability of learned behaviors, and better coverage of open-ended task domains. The concepts of developmental learning are well-suited for the curiosity-driven, playful, explorative learning using simple toys that one does not have to know a lot about and where action failures are unproblematic.

6.1.3 Hybrid Knowledge Representation and Reasoning for Cognition-Enabled Robots

The realization of computational models for accomplishing everyday manipulation tasks for any object and any purpose would be a disruptive breakthrough in the creation of versatile, general-purpose robot agents; and it is a grand challenge for AI and robotics. Humans are able to accomplish tasks such as "cut up the fruit" for many types of fruit by generating a large variety of context-specific manipulation behaviors. They can typically accomplish the tasks on the first attempt despite uncertain physical conditions and novel objects. Acting so effectively requires comprehensive reasoning about the possible consequences of intended behavior before physically interacting with the real world.

Our research hypothesis is that a knowledge representation and reasoning (KR&R) framework based on explicitly-represented and machine-interpretable inner-world models can enable robots to contextualize underdetermined manipulation task requests on the first attempt. For this purpose the robot needs a hybrid symbolic/subsymbolic KR&R framework that will contextualize actions by reasoning symbolically in an abstract and generalized manner but also by reasoning with "one's eyes and hands" through mental simulation and imagistic reasoning. This requires three breakthrough research results:

1. modeling and parameterization of manipulation motion patterns and understanding the resulting effects under uncertain conditions,
2. the ability to mentally simulate imagined and observed manipulation tasks to link them to the robot's knowledge and experience and,
3. the on-demand acquisition of task-specific causal models for novel manipulation tasks through mental physics-based simulations.

The main societal impact of these breakthrough results will be the improvement of cognitive capabilities for explainable, robust, and trustworthy robot control programs that can accomplish a broad spectrum of service tasks and thereby substantially advance the field of human assistant robotics.

6.1.4 Everyday Activity Science and Engineering

In the collaborative research center EASE ("Everyday Activity Science and Engineering," https://ease-crc.org/) we investigate the design, realization, and analysis of information processing models that enable robot agents (and humans) to master manipulation tasks that may appear simple and routine, but that are, in fact, complex and demanding.

EASE takes the perspective that the mastery of everyday activity can be formulated as the computational problem of deciding how robots have to move their bodies in order to accomplish underspecified manipulation tasks and that these decisions should be based on knowledge and reasoning.

The unique approach that EASE takes is that we investigate and develop complete robot agents that perform end-to-end context-driven manipulation tasks by leveraging

1. explicitly-represented knowledge,
2. explicit inherently-adaptable generalized action plans and,
3. powerful prospection mechanisms based on machine-understandable inner-world models.

The core of our approach lies in designing, building, and analyzing generative models for accomplishing everyday household tasks. A generative model provides the basis for a mapping from the desired outcomes of a task to the motion parameter values that are most likely to succeed in generating these outcomes. Such a model can be viewed as a joint distribution of motion parameter values and the corresponding task outcomes. In EASE, the generative model is realized through knowledge representation and reasoning, which is based on the robot's tightly-coupled symbolic and subsymbolic knowledge about the tasks it is performing, the objects it is acting on, and the environment in which it is operating. These generative models are used to simulate various task execution candidate strategies before committing to one particular strategy to be performed in the physical world.

The research into generative models of everyday activities is inspired by investigations of the manner in which humans master their everyday manipulation tasks, the results of which provide the computational mechanisms that can then be used to replicate these human abilities in cognitive robots. EASE not only investigates action selection and control but also the methods needed to acquire the knowledge, skills, and competence required for flexible, reliable, and efficient mastery of these activities. *Competence* means that robot agents are able to translate underdetermined action requests into the appropriate behaviors and adapt their behaviors spontaneously to new situations and demands, allowing them to assist humans reliably in a wide variety of settings. Robots will have to act fluently without hesitation, understand what they are doing, communicate the reasons for their choice of behaviors, and improve performance by learning from experience, by reading, by observing, or by playing. Performing actions flexibly, robustly, and competently requires intuitive physics and commonsense reasoning in order to translate desired effects into the motion parameterizations that can achieve them.

EASE selects everyday activities as its target domain because they allow robots

1. to structure their activities such that they exhibit regularities that can be exploited for better performance,
2. to continually acquire readily actionable commonsense and intuitive physics knowledge and,

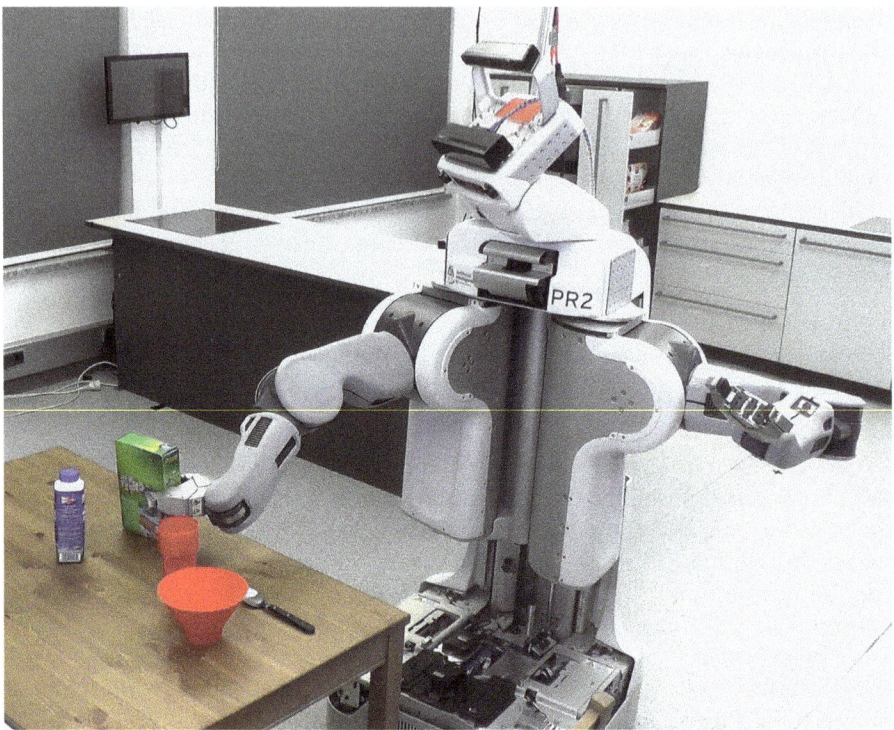

Fig. 6.1 PR2 robot setting a table in the EASE Household Marathon Experiment

3. to improve performance by specializing general actions through the exploitation of task constraints, structure, and regularities.

In the EASE *Robot Household Marathon Experiment* (Kazhoyan et al., 2021, https://www.youtube.com/watch?v=pv_n9FQRoZQ&t=44s) we demonstrated a generative model which enables physical robot agents to set and clean a table given vague task requests. This generative model only requires a carefully designed, generalized action plan for fetching and placing objects, which is autonomously contextualized by the model for each individual object transportation task. Thus, the robot autonomously infers the body motion that achieves the respective object transportation task and avoids unwanted side effects (e.g., knocking over a glass when placing a spoon on the table) depending on the type and state of the object to be transported (be it a spoon, bowl, cereal box, milk box, or mug), the original location (be it the drawer, the high drawer, or the table), and the task context (be it setting or cleaning the table, loading the dishwasher, or throwing away items). The body motions generated to perform the actions are varied and complex and, when required, include subactions such as opening and closing containers, as well as coordinated, bimanual manipulation tasks (Fig. 6.1).

We were able to show that the competence of the generative model can be increased by asserting additional generalized domain, commonsense, and intuitive physics knowledge and reasoning, and that substantial parts of such knowledge can be acquired by the robot itself through experience, observation, and taking advice. In addition, the model exhibits impressive introspective capabilities that enable the robot agents employing it to answer questions about what they are doing, why, how, what they expect to happen, and so on. In simulation, we accomplished this scenario in even more variations, such as different kitchen setups with different furniture arrangements, on different robot platforms, and we also applied our generalized fetch and place plan in different domains, specifically retail and assembly domains.

Our future research will focus on the integration of our approach to parametrized general planning and the hybrid KR&R framework into a general cognitive architecture for autonomous robots. On the basis of this architecture we will design, implement, and experimentally investigate robots that can successfully interact with other robots and with humans in virtual and physical environments. This involves a transition from a focus on goals, intentions, and actions, to shared goals, shared intentions, and joint action, requiring the use of powerful mechanisms such as implicit communication.

6.2 Communication with Robots

The expert responses also reflect the challenge of enabling communication with robots.[1] We formulated 11 items on human–robot communication in everyday life, all looking ahead to 2030. Will robots then tend to replace humans situationally in interpersonal communication? Will specialized robots then provide psychological advice (counseling)? Will humans then trust AI more than humans themselves? Will AI assist in rational choice (guidance)? Will humans first seek a doctor's advice from a robot in telemedicine (consultation)? As detailed elsewhere (Engel & Dahlhaus, 2022, p. 358, Table 20.A2), the answer to all these questions is *probably not*. While the expert group is thus quite pessimistic about robots providing required guidance, counseling, and consultation, the group appears *undecided* if it comes to communication with personal avatars. In this regard, it appears only *possible* that lifelogging will issue in communication of humans with personal avatars, and such avatars will have become steady advisory life companions. The same undecided tendency characterizes the response to the statement that robots keep lonely people of different ages company at home. In contrast, three scenarios appear *rather likely than unlikely*. So, the group of experts expects that robots will keep older people company at home,

---

[1] Overall assessments. The initial report on the project documents (Engel, 2020) group-specific statistics (for social science vs. STEM disciplines vs. stakeholders in politics). Chapter 3 of this volume provides further study details.

that bots will communicate as well as humans, and that AI and robots take up increasingly more assistant functions in the life of humans.[2]

6.2.1 The Challenge of Enabling Robotic Skills

At first glance, the opinions the experts expressed in these answers turn out to be quite pessimistic. On the one hand, this may be because sample tasks, such as counseling, guidance, and consultation, require ambitious functional and extra-functional (cognitive and emotional) skills, such as empathy, and they do not assume that robots will already have them in the survey's reference year, 2030. On the other hand, the answers can also reflect the difficulty that potential users need not accept a robot simply because it appears to be competent. We want to shed light on both aspects. While in this section we ask about the temporal perspective on realizing a broad spectrum of robotic skills, in the following section, we aim to shed light on the question of user acceptance.

We formulated the survey question as follows: "The technical development of AI includes the solution of highly complex tasks. By when, do you suspect, will AI have the following capabilities?" The response scale follows:

1. is already possible
2. by 2025
3. by 2030
4. by 2035
5. by 2040
6. by 2045
7. by 2050
8. later
9. will not be possible at all

Figure 6.2 shows a wide range in the mean expected time periods and considerable uncertainty in the underlying temporal estimates. Regarding the functions expected only in the longer term, the temporal estimates exhibit a particularly large spread. Table 6.1 explains which functions are graphed in each case.

Confirmatory factor analysis of these temporal estimates suggests the grouping that the left column of Table 6.1 indicates. Even if usable for a first orientation only, the CFA suggests a relatively clear pattern of relations *between these assessments.* Skills B, C, and D constitute a first factor that appears to cover robotic self-control and motor skills, associated with carrying out physical tasks *on people* autonomously, and moving around in the rooms of an apartment *like a human.* The factor

---

[2] We analyzed the relationships between these expert ratings by a factor analysis of the polychoric correlations involved. The online appendix to this chapter at https://github.com/viewsandinsights/AI documents the results.

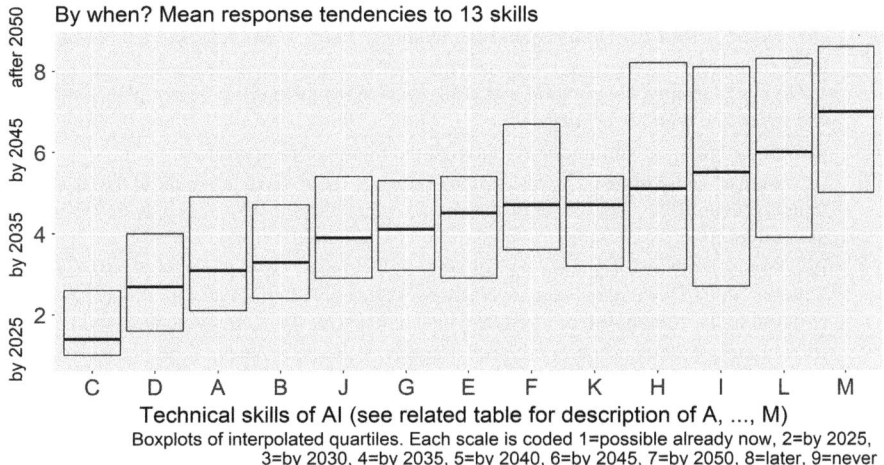

Fig. 6.2 Robotic skills: By when?

correlates highly ($r = 0.71$) with a second factor. The skills A, J, and K constitute this second factor, also covering aspects of robotic self-control and motor skills, this time regarding autonomously moving in space and performing physical tasks. Striking here is the larger time spread between the single functions. With G, E, and F, the next factor represents cognitive abilities necessary to conduct personal conversations. Finally, a factor that appears to indicate cognitive and creative skills *like a human's* covers the last four skills, H, I, L, and M. Thus, by and large, we observe a sequence in which robotic self-control and motor skills come first and cognitive functions come next.

6.2.2 Expected Robotic Skills and the Challenge of Communication with Robots

Robotic assistance implies repeated encounters, several times a day over a long period of time. This leads us to expect that accepting such encounters will only occur if they are sufficiently pleasant. This is challenging in two ways. On the one hand, robots must become equipped with the necessary motor, cognitive, and communicative skills, and on the other hand, people must be able to imagine interacting with intelligent machines. Interacting with a robot implies communicating with it. But that is exactly what people cannot quite imagine today. The results in Chap. 1 show that people today still find it very difficult to imagine conversations with robots.[3]

---

[3] Similarly, Stubbe et al. (2019, p. 8) cite a study on the question of how humans and robots should divide their work in different areas of activity in the future. As the cited source at statista.com

Table 6.1 The technical skills of AI graphed in Fig. 6.2

A^2	Drones can deliver mail and parcels reliably and securely to any recipient address in cities.
B^1	Robots can autonomously carry out activities in the care of people in need of care. Example 1: Giving bedridden people food and drink (feed, have them drink from a glass), raise the bed to eat and then lower it again.
C^1	Robots can navigate autonomously through the rooms of an apartment.
D^1	In a room of an apartment, robots can, for example, move toward people in the same way (quickly, carefully, ...) or move away from them in the same way as people do among themselves.
E^3	Robots can autonomously carry out activities in the care of people in need of care. Example 2: Being able to have personal conversations with people in need of care in a personalized (tailored to the person, learned from the interaction with her) communication style.
F^3	Robots can autonomously carry out activities in the care of people in need of care. Example 3: Being able to hold personal conversations with people in need of care that relate to one another, in terms of content (being able to follow up on previous conversation content).
G^3	Robots can infer underlying behavioral intentions from observing verbal and extraverbal human behavior.
H^4	The reference data sets available for training robots are as extensive as the wealth of biographical experience that people typically learn.
I^4	Robots program themselves.
J^2	Autonomous driving is safe and reliable in cities.
K^2	Assistant robots can take over household tasks, such as preparing food, setting and clearing the table, operating the dishwasher and washing machine, and loading and unloading them.
L^4	Like humans, robots can transfer solution ideas from one problem area to another.
M^4	When the experience to solve a problem is lacking, "common sense" may offer a second-best solution. Robots are now also able to develop a contextual understanding of a problem.

Grouped according to the CFA reported in the online appendix to this chapter: 1 Robotic self-control and motor skills, 1: Carry out physical tasks *on people* autonomously and move around in the rooms of an apartment *like a human*; 2 Robotic self-control and motor skills, 2: Move autonomously in space and perform physical tasks; 3 Cognition, 1: Cognitive abilities to conduct personal conversations; 4 Cognition, 2: Cognitive & creative skills like a human.

Analogously, we also see in the present context that communicative skills are primarily not expected from an assistant robot. On the contrary, for a large majority of respondents to our population survey, assistant robots should not even have the ability to conduct personal conversations. Taken together, this creates a complicated situation. The reason is a remarkable correlation between the scales *talk* and *care* that we introduced in Chap. 1. "Talk" reflects the personal readiness to have conversations with robots, and "care" reflects the readiness to have robots assist in one's care. Both scales are strongly correlated ($r = 0.66$) and indicate that the stronger the

---

reports, the online survey was fielded from October 2017 to May 2018, with ca. 11,000 respondents. Like the present study, that one assigned robots the communication function to a very small extent too. The cited source reports these figures: Communication and teamwork (4% vs. 73%), decision-making (8% vs. 48%), creativity and problem-solving (9% vs. 39%), repetitive activities (39% vs. 17%), and physically strenuous activities (70% vs. 6%) for "robot alone" vs. "human alone" (each difference to 100%: "human and robot together").

Table 6.2 Expected skills of care robots

Item wording	Figure 6.3	Yes[a]	Other[b]	No[c]
An assistant robot should be able to ...		Row percent		
... have trivial everyday conversations with someone in need of care to pass the time	Everyday conversation	35.90	32.82	31.28
... have personal or very personal conversations with someone in need of care	Personal conversation	8.12	18.78	73.10
... play card games, board games, or the like with someone in need of care to pass the time	Play card/ board games	69.04	19.80	11.17
... pick up and take away items for someone in need of care	Pick up/take away items	96.53	0.99	2.48
... maintain (emergency) contact with treating doctors, nurses, and family members for a person in need of care	(emergency) contacts	76.92	8.72	14.36
... help a person in need of care to put on and take off clothes	Dress up and off	57.73	13.92	28.35
... assist a person in need of care with personal hygiene	Help with pers. hygiene	46.70	17.26	36.04
... give a person in need of care food (feed, give to drink)	Feed, give to drink	51.76	18.59	29.65
... pay attention to the intake of medication	Monitor: Medication	69.95	11.82	18.23

Percentage base of survey-weighted frequency distributions: $N_k = 194$ to 203 (excl. "don't-know")
[a] An assistant robot should be specially trained for this
[b] An assistant robot should rather be trained for other tasks
[c] An assistant robot should not be able to do this

readiness is in one respect, the stronger the readiness is in the other. Conversely, with no willingness to communicate with robots, there is no willingness to include care robots in one's life if necessary. The present section takes up these two scales and relates them to the qualification profile of an assistant robot as it emerges from the respondents' preferences.

We worded the survey question this way: "Provided that an assistant robot would later be able to perform the following tasks competently, reliably, and without errors: For what types of activities and conversations with people in need of care should an assistant robot be specially trained? What kind of conversations and activities should remain taboo for an assistant robot?" This was followed by the items Table 6.2 displays. For each such item, respondents were asked to choose between the three responses, the graphs of whose distributions Fig. 6.3 shows:

- "An assistant robot should be specially trained for this" (bottom left [0] to top [1.0])
- "An assistant robot should rather be trained for other tasks" (top [0] to bottom right [1.0]) and
- "An assistant robot should not be able to do this" (bottom right [0] to bottom left [1.0]).

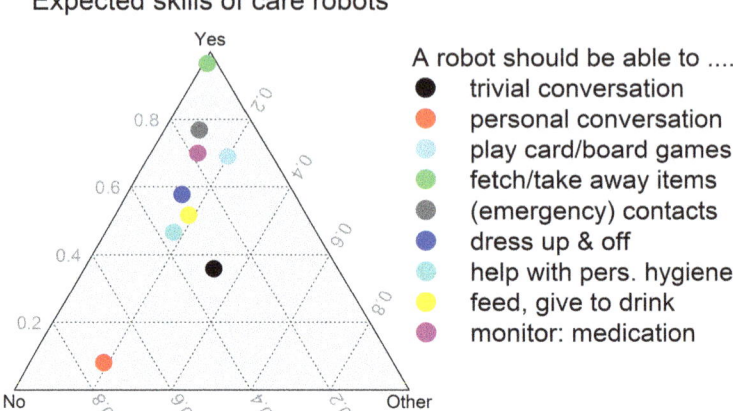

Fig. 6.3 Expected skills of care robots

By locating each skill in the triangle of these three answers, the graphic conveys a good impression of the polarization pattern of the involved skills. The items form a narrow band along the no-yes poles; only one item (i.e., everyday conversation) has a value greater than 0.2 for the response option "Other." Nearly all respondents prefer picking up and taking away items, only 2.5% would ban that skill. Shares between 0.6 and 0.8 preferred three further skills, while at the same time shares of less than 0.2 banned them. This applies to maintaining (emergency) contacts, monitoring medication, and playing cards/board games. The pronounced reverse of this high/low pattern holds for personal conversation that few approved and many rejected. The personal and everyday communication skills are the two skills that reach lowest acceptance and, at the same time, highest and third-highest rejection.

How does the preferred qualification profile of assistant robots correlate with the respondents' willingness to talk with them and to use them as care robots? To find this out, we use the scales of factor scores *talk* and *care* that we introduced in Chap. 1 and correlate them with the robotic skills the present section considers.[4] The analysis shows that whether someone thinks that an assistant robot should be trained for a special task or not depends sometimes less and sometimes more on personal readiness. For instance, the "pick up and take away items" as well as the maintenance of "(emergency) contacts" correlate least with both *talk* and *care*. Personal readiness then makes only a small difference. The situation is different with "help with personal hygiene," for which we observe a small correlation with *talk* (0.26) and a high correlation with *care* (0.61). Thus, assistance robots receive this task primarily from respondents who can imagine using the services of a care robot for

---

[4] Due to the combination of (nominal, metric) scale levels involved, a dummy regression analysis appeared most appropriate to compute the relevant multiple R's. Table A4 in the Online appendix to this chapter at https://github.com/viewsandinsights/AI reports the results of the 18 linear dummy regressions. Here, we focus on its entries in the columns labeled b_{yes} and R.

themselves or a close relative. Therefore, the skills we expect of an assistant robot are partly quite independent of personal readiness and partly depend upon it. This also applies to communication skills: both skills, everyday and personal conversation, correlate moderately-to-strongly with the *personal* willingness to *talk* and *care*.

6.2.3 Correlates of Talk and Care with Pictures of Robots

To make it easier for the interviewees to get started in the interview, we wanted to know what they associate with the term *robot*. We presented 12 pictures showing different types of robots and asked, "When the language comes up with 'robots': With what do you spontaneously associate with this term?"[5] *Pepper* makes it to number 1, probably due to its frequent media presence. It also comes as no surprise that a typical industrial robot also frequently makes it into the TOP 3 preference set. *PR2* from EASE and the *Care-O-bot 4* service robot from Fraunhofer IPA also often correspond to the spontaneously expected image of a robot.

Most of the 12 pictures of robots presented to the respondents do not correlate with *talk* or *care*. Of the nine machine-like robots, only the care robot "Service-Assistant" from Fraunhofer IPA shows weak but statistically significant correlations with these scales (talk: $r = 0.21$, b/s.e = 3.0; care: $r = 0.29$, b/s.e = 4.1). Regarding the three robots with suggested human-like physical attributes (head and arms), two correlate with *talk* but not with *care*: Fraunhofer IPA's "Care-O-bot 4" ($r = 0.22$; b/s.e = 3.2) and the popular "Pepper" ($r = 0.14$, b/s.e = 2.1).

How People Perceive Social Robots

Intended as an easy entry to the survey, the above correlation analysis represents rather a coincidental by-product than a systematic exploration into the physical attractiveness of robots. However, we can refer to reviews and other studies. For instance, following Bartneck et al. (2020), the humans' inclination toward anthropomorphism is likely to assign assistance robots to the role of digital companions in daily interaction (Bartneck et al., 2020). Lum (2020, pp. 145–146) discusses human–robot interaction "outside of industrial and manufacturing of products" and underlines the sociability of robots as "becoming an increasingly important component that robots may need in order to interact in a human world." She also stresses the need "to focus on anthropomorphism directly" and concludes from her review that "one of the main challenges when designing robots will be people's acceptance of robots sharing their daily lives" (Lum, 2020, p. 148). Stroessner (2020) identifies three dimensions in the perception of robot faces—warmth, competence, and discomfort—and reviews findings that underline the relevance of gender-typicality and humanlike vs. machinelike faces, in terms of evaluative responses and contact desirability with such faces (Stroessner, 2020, p. 38). Liu et al. (2022) present a

---

[5] Along with all references involved, the complete list of robots, along with their individual rankings, appears in the online appendix to this chapter at https://github.com/viewsandinsights/AI

recent study on people's perceptions of social robots. They examine "how appearance and characteristic narrative, combined with warmth and competence perceptions, impact people's perceptions and acceptance of robots" (p. 324), and, for instance, found out that "competent robots are preferred over warm robots, and appearance design is more effective than a characteristic narrative" (Liu et al., 2022, p. 338).

Human–Robot Interaction in Care and Daily Life
The development of assistance robots, especially for use near humans, poses a major challenge in various respects. Enabling cognitive functions and a well-functioning interplay of cognitive, communicative, and motor skills places high demands on the art of programming and robot construction. In addition, there are design questions to solve. Robots may have very different shapes, look machine-like or human-like, convey a warm and competent impression, trigger positive reactions or feelings of discomfort. Accordingly, people may find it not always desirable to interact and communicate with such robots. And given the current lack of willingness to hold conversations with robots, the solution of design issues may be a great help in the further development of assistance robots. In the nature of things, we will best achieve this through interdisciplinary cooperation of robotics, cognition science, psychology, and sociology.

Acknowledgments The research reported in this chapter has been partially supported by the German Research Foundation DFG, as part of Collaborative Research Center (Sonderforschungsbereich) 1320 "EASE—Everyday Activity Science and Engineering," University of Bremen (http://www.ease-crc.org/).

References

Bartneck, C., Belpaeme, T., Eyssel, F., Kanda, T., Keijsers, M., & Sabanovic, S. (2020). *Human-robot interaction: An introduction*. Cambridge University Press.

Berner, C., Brockman, G., Chan, B., Cheung, V., Debiak, P., Dennison, C., Farhi, D., Fischer, Q., Hashme, S., Hesse, C., Józefowicz, R., Gray, S., Olsson, C., Pachocki, J., Petrov, M., Pinto, H. D. O., Raiman, J., Salimans, T., Schlatter, J., Schneider, J., Sidor, S., Sutskever, I., Tang, J., Wolski, F., & Zhang, S. (2019). *Dota 2 with large scale deep reinforcement learning*. Retrieved January 16, 2022, from https://arxiv.org/abs/1912.06680

Craik, K. (1943). *The nature of explanation*. University Press.

Engel, U. (2020). *Blick in die Zukunft. Wie künstliche Intelligenz das Leben verändern wird. Universität Bremen* [View in the future. How artificial intelligence will change life]. Retrieved January 13, 2022, from https://www.viewsandinsights.com/fileadmin/bilder/referenzen/ki-delphi-ergebnisse.pdf

Engel, U., & Dahlhaus, L. (2022). Data quality and privacy concerns in digital trace data. In U. Engel, A. Quan-Haase, S. Liu, & L. Lyberg (Eds.), *Handbook of computational social science, Vol. 1 - Theory, case studies and ethics* (pp. 343–362). Routledge. https://doi.org/10.4324/9781003024583-23

Jeannerod, M. (2001). Neural simulation of action: A unifying mechanism for motor cognition. *NeuroImage, 14*(1), S103–S109. Retrieved January 16, 2022, from https://www.sciencedirect.com/science/article/pii/S1053811901908328

Kazhoyan, G., Stelter, S., Kenfack, F. K., Koralewski, S., & Beetz, M. (2021). *2021 IEEE International Conference on Robotics and Automation (ICRA)* (pp. 9382–9388). IEEE. https://doi.org/10.1109/ICRA48506.2021.9560774

Kuipers, B., Feigenbaum, E., Hart, P., & Shakey, N. N. (2017). From conception to history. *AI Magazine, 38*(1), 88–103.

Laird, J. E., Gluck, K., Anderson, J., Forbus, K. D., Jenkins, O. C., Lebiere, C., Salvucci, D., Scheutz, M., Thomaz, A., Trafton, G., Wray, R. E., Mohan, S., & Kirk, J. R. (2017). Interactive task learning. *IEEE Intelligent Systems, 32*(4), 6–21. https://doi.org/10.1109/MIS.2017.3121552

Lake, B. M., Ullman, T. D., Tenenbaum, J. B., & Gershman, S. (2016). Building machines that learn and think like people. *The Behavioral and Brain Sciences, 40*.

Levine, S., Pastor, P., Krizhevsky, A., Ibarz, J., & Quillen, D. (2018). Learning hand-eye coordination for robotic grasping with deep learning and large-scale data collection. *The International Journal of Robotics Research, 37*(4–5), 421–436. https://doi.org/10.1177/0278364917710318

Liu, S. X., Arredondo, E., Mieczkowski, H., Hancock, J., & Reeves, B. (2022). A picture is (still) worth a thousand words. The impact of appearance and characteristic narratives on people's perceptions of social robots. In U. Engel, A. Quan-Haase, S. Liu, & L. Lyberg (Eds.), *Handbook of computational social science, Vol. 1 - Theory, case studies and ethics* (pp. 324–342). Routledge.

Lum, H. C. (2020). The role of consumer robots in our everyday lives. In R. Pak, E. J. de Visser, & E. Rovira (Eds.), *Living with robots* (pp. 141–152). Academic Press. https://doi.org/10.1016/B978-0-12-815367-3.00007-4

Marcus, G. (2020). *The next decade in AI: Four steps towards robust artificial intelligence. CoRR, abs/2002.06177*. Retrieved January 16, 2022, from https://arxiv.org/abs/2002.06177

Marcus, G., & Davis, E. (2021). Insights for AI from the human mind. *Communications of the ACM, 64*(1), 38–41.

McDermott, D. (1992). Robot planning. *AI Magazine, 13*(2), 55–79.

Mnih, V., Kavukcuoglu, K., Silver, D., Rusu, A. A., Veness, J., Bellemare, M. G., Graves, A., Riedmiller, M., Fidjeland, A. K., Ostrovski, G., Petersen, S., Beattie, C., Sadik, A., Antonoglou, J., King, H., Kumaran, D., Wierstra, D., Legg, S., & Hassabis, D. (2015). Human-level control through deep reinforcement learning. *Nature, 518*, 529–533. https://doi.org/10.1038/nature14236

Nau, D., Ghallab, M., & Traverso, P. (2004). *Automated planning: Theory & practice*. Morgan Kaufmann Publishers.

OpenAI, Akkaya, I., Andrychowicz, M., Chociej, M., Litwin, M., McGrew, B., Petron, A., Paino, A., Plappert, M., Powell, G., Ribas, R., Schneider, J., Tezak, N., Tworek, J., Welinder, P., Weng, L., Yuan, Q., Zaremba, W., & Zhang, L. (2019). *Solving Rubik's cube with a robot hand*. Retrieved January 16, 2022, from https://arxiv.org/pdf/1910.07113.pdf

Rule, J., Tenenbaum, J., & Piantadosi, S. (2020). The child as hacker. *Trends in Cognitive Sciences, 24*, 900–915.

Schrittwieser, J., Antonoglou, I., Hubert, T., Simonyan, K., Sifre, L., Schmitt, S., Guez, A., Lockhart, E., Hassabis, D., Graepel, T., Lillicrap, T. P., & Silver, D. (2019). *Mastering atari, go, chess and shogi by planning with a learned model. CoRR, abs/1911.08265*. Retrieved January 16, 2022, from http://arxiv.org/abs/1911.08265

Schwettmann, S., Tenenbaum, J., & Kanwisher, N. (2018, January). *Evidence for an intuitive physics engine in the human brain*.

Shanahan, M. (2006). A cognitive architecture that combines internal simulation with a global workspace. *Consciousness and Cognition, 15*(2), 433–449. Retrieved January 16, 2022, from http://www.sciencedirect.com/science/article/pii/S1053810005001510

Silver, D., Huang, A., Maddison, C. J., Guez, A., Sifre, L., Driessche, G., Schrittwieser, J., Antonoglou, I., Panneershelvam, V., Lanctot, M., Dieleman, S., Grewe, D., Nham, J., Kalchbrenner, N., Sutskever, I., Lillicrap, T., Leach, M., Kavukcuoglu, K., Graepel, T., &

Hassabis, D. (2016). Mastering the game of Go with deep neural networks and tree search. *Nature, 529*(7587), 484–489. https://doi.org/10.1038/nature16961

Silver, D., Schrittwieser, J., Simonyan, K., Antonoglou, I., Huang, A., Guez, A., Hubert, T., Baker, L., Lai, M., Bolton, A., Chen, Y., Lillicrap, T., Hui, F., Sifre, L., Driessche, G., Graepel, T., & Hassabis, D. (2017). Mastering the game of Go without human knowledge. *Nature, 550*(7676), 354–359.

Spelke, E. (2000). Core knowledge. *The American Psychologist, 55,* 1233–1243.

Spelke, E., & Kinzler, K. (2009). Innateness, learning, and rationality. *Child Development Perspectives, 3,* 96–98.

Stroessner, S. J. (2020). On the social perception of robots: Measurement, moderation, and implications. In R. Pak, E. J. de Visser, & E. Rovira (Eds.), *Living with robots* (pp. 21–47). Academic Press. https://doi.org/10.1016/B978-0-12-815367-3.00002-5

Stubbe, J., Mock, J., & Wischmann, S. (2019). *Akzeptanz von Servicerobotern: Tools und Strategien für den erfolgreichen betrieblichen Einsatz. Begleitforschung PAiCE. [Acceptance of service robots: Tools and strategies for successful operational use].* Retrieved January 07, 2022, from https://www.iit-berlin.de/publikation/akzeptanz-von-servicerobotern-tools-und-strategien-fuer-den-erfolgreichen-betrieblichen-einsatz/

Szpunar, K. K., Spreng, R. N., & Schacter, D. L. (2014). A taxonomy of prospection: Introducing an organizational framework for future-oriented cognition. *PNAS Proceedings of the National Academy of Sciences of the United States of America, 111*(52), 18414–18421. https://doi.org/10.1073/pnas.1417144111

Ullman, T., & Tenenbaum, J. (2020). Bayesian models of conceptual development: Learning as building models of the world. *Annual Review of Developmental Psychology, 2,* 533–558.

Ullman, T., Spelke, E., Battaglia, P., & Tenenbaum, J. (2017). Mind games: Game engines as an architecture for intuitive physics. *Trends in Cognitive Sciences, 21.*

Vernon, D. (2014). *Artificial cognitive systems: A primer.* MIT Press.

Williams, D. (2018). *The mind as a predictive modelling engine: Generative models, structural similarity, and mental representation.* PhD thesis.

Wolpert, D. (2011). *The real reason for brains.* TEDGlobal 2011. Retrieved from https://www.ted.com/talks/daniel_wolpert_the_real_reason_for_brains/discussion

Michael Beetz is a professor for Computer Science at the Faculty for Mathematics & Informatics of the University of Bremen and a head of the Institute for Artificial Intelligence (IAI). IAI investigates AI-based control methods for robotic agents, with a focus on human-scale everyday manipulation tasks. He is the coordinator of the German Collaborative Research Centre EASE (Everyday Activity Science and Engineering). His research interests include plan-based control of robotic agents, knowledge processing and representation for robots, integrated robot learning, and cognitive perception.

Uwe Engel is a Professor at the University of Bremen (Germany), where he held a chair in sociology from 2000 until his retirement in autumn 2020. In 2007, he founded the Social Science Methods Centre of Bremen University, and directed this institution until 2020. Current work focuses on computational social science and human–robot interaction. See https://www.viewsandinsights.com/en/welcome-to-views-insights and https://orcid.org/0000-0001-8420-9677 for details.

Hagen Langer is a senior researcher at the Institute for Artificial Intelligence at the University of Bremen. His research interests include natural language processing, knowledge representation, multiagent systems, cognitive robotics, and machine learning. He received a doctoral degree from Georg-August-Universität Göttingen and he also holds a habilitation from the University of Osnabrück. Since 2017, he is the managing director of the Collaborative Research Center EASE—Everyday Activity Science and Engineering (http://www.ease-crc.org).

Open Access This chapter is licensed under the terms of the Creative Commons Attribution 4.0 International License (http://creativecommons.org/licenses/by/4.0/), which permits use, sharing, adaptation, distribution and reproduction in any medium or format, as long as you give appropriate credit to the original author(s) and the source, provide a link to the Creative Commons license and indicate if changes were made.

The images or other third party material in this chapter are included in the chapter's Creative Commons license, unless indicated otherwise in a credit line to the material. If material is not included in the chapter's Creative Commons license and your intended use is not permitted by statutory regulation or exceeds the permitted use, you will need to obtain permission directly from the copyright holder.

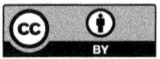

Chapter 7
Ethical Challenges of Assistive Robotics in the Elderly Care: Review and Reflection

Mona Abdel-Keream

Abstract Over the last decade, the range of robotic applications in the healthcare sector has expanded rapidly. These applications can range from dispensing medication to providing more personalized services to caretakers. However, this kind of robotization is associated with severe ethical and societal implications. To advance the design and acceptability of socially interactive robots it is, therefore, necessary to consider and analyze those concerns. The RoPHa research project aims at supporting care-dependent people to lead more independent life. This chapter examines potential ethical challenges and impacts in elderly care that were discussed during the design of the robotic system in the project. For evaluating the effect of assistive robotics on elderly care in practice, the MEESTAR model was applied. The ethical implications of the proposed applications were mapped to seven moral dimensions, such as autonomy, justice, privacy, etc. Each dimension were examined from three different perspectives (individual, organizational, and societal). All identified ethical implications were graded based on the degree of ethical justifiability. The results include ethically relevant questions regarding the role of the robotic system, its technical implications, economic and distrust barriers, occupational safety, data security as well as the legal and safety responsibilities of all involved parties.

Keywords Elderly care · Ethics · Assitive Robotics · MEESTAR

7.1 Introduction

RoPHa: Robots for the Support of Older People and People in Need of Care
Against the backdrop of the demographic development in Germany and other western societies, the support of older people and people in need of care is standard in discussing possible applications for robots. For the year 2050, it is projected,

---

M. Abdel-Keream (✉)
University of Bremen, Bremen, Germany
e-mail: abdelker@uni-bremen.de

according to the latest report of Eurostat (Eurostat, 2020), that their relative share of the total population will gradually increase to reach 29.4%.

The *RoPHa*[1] (*Ro*buste *P*erzeption für die interaktive Unterstützung älterer Nutzer bei *Ha*ndhabungsaufgaben im häuslichen Umfeld) project—funded by the Federal Ministry of Education and Research (Bundesministerium für Bildung und Forschung, BMBF) aims at supporting care-dependent people to lead and maintain a longer independent life especially in the context of food consumption. The assistive robot should not only aid in preparing meals but should also assist the caretaker in consuming their meal. Since older adults face serious nutrition concerns and deficits, food intake is a practical application for a robotic system. The overall objective is to enhance the capabilities of interactive assistance robots to safely perform everyday manipulation tasks in complex and dynamic environments. The developed technologies were implemented and demonstrated on the Care-O-bot® 4[2] service robot. Together with experts from the care sector, different use cases were defined including preparing and serving food to the patient.

To advance the design and acceptability of socially interactive robots, it is necessary to discuss these issues' ethical, societal, and legal perspectives. The MEESTAR model (Manzeschke et al., 2015) was used to evaluate ethical implications of the envisioned technical assistance systems. This instrument was specifically designed to provide an ethical evaluation of socio-technical arrangements. It determines the impact of such arrangements concerning their design and functionality based on concrete scenarios. The evaluation aided in the identification of ethically relevant problems as well as in the joint development of proposed solutions.

7.2 Methodology

7.2.1 User Case Definition

The MEESTAR model requires a representative description of the technical system. The description of the system is provided through graphical sketches and diagrams. The description was formulated as detailed as possible with various design variables in mind to achieve a reliable system assessment. The provided description was regarded as an initial version of the system. The assessment process is then continually reiterated as more profound knowledge regarding aspects and features of the system and its environment, including users and other participants, becomes available.

For the initial system description, a care needs assessment was conducted through organizing preliminary observations in three facilities of the "Stiftung evangelische Altenheim." They provide different forms of nursing care services, including

---

[1] https://www.ropha-projekt.de/ [accessed on 12th of Jan, 2022].

[2] https://www.care-o-bot.de/en/care-o-bot-4.html [accessed on 12th of Jan, 2022].

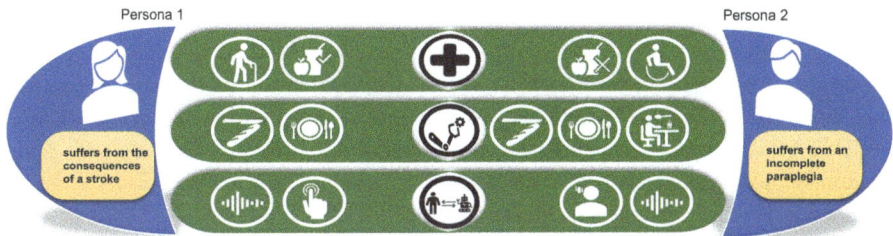

Fig. 7.1 Definition of the personas in RoPHa with different requirement profiles. While Persona 1 requires a walking aid for locomotion but can still eat independently, Persona 2 can only get around with an electric wheelchair due to incomplete paraplegia. Persona 2, therefore, requires additional help with food consumption. The last bar lists the possible interaction modalities (voice input, tablet application, head button on the wheelchair)

daycare, young care, and care of persons who have dementia. The assessment aided in identifying the needs and unmet needs of people requiring care and the current support already provided for them. This initial assesment aided in defining desirable assistive functionalities of a robotic system. Based on the preliminary observation on the side, two personas (see Fig.7.1) were identified as potential users of the robotic assistance solution.

One persona suffers from the consequences of a stroke (hemiparesis). She can still eat independently but has difficulties with fine motor skills. The second persona suffers from incomplete paraplegia from the cervical spine onward and is therefore no longer able to eat independently. Based on the proximity of the robot to the user, the RoPHa project defined three key assistive functionalities, including practical tasks:

- "Preparatory tasks," e.g.:
  - Setting the table
  - Warming food
  - Cleaning the table

- "Assistance at the table," e.g.:
  - Cutting food
  - Opening a bottle
  - Pouring drinks

- "Direct interaction," e.g.:
  - Serving food
  - Serving drinks

7.2.2 Ethical Evaluation

To consider all relevant implications, the ethical evaluation of the system requires the expertise of multiple disciplines. In the form of an interdisciplinary workshop, MEESTAR provides a reference framework to structure discussions about system-related ethical aspects with respect to a set of pre-defined dimensions, as outlined below and graphed in Manzeschke et al. (2015, p. 14).

Since MEESTAR seeks to determine and evaluate the ethical implications of socio-technical arrangements using concrete scenarios, a description of the system, including the intended context of use, was presented to all workshop participants. Three interdisciplinary working groups were formed, consisting of members of the research groups involved in the project and the pilot users. Each group reflected on and analyzed the case study from one of the three levels of observation mentioned in MEESTAR:

- individual (IL)
- social (SL)
- organizational (OL)

The first step focused on the identification of ethical problems and challenges. The technical assistance system was assessed regarding the seven ethical evaluation dimensions named in MEESTAR:

1. Care
2. Autonomy
3. Security
4. Justice
5. Privacy
6. Participation
7. Self-Perception

In addition, the identified ethical problems and areas of conflict were hierarchized into four levels in terms of their severity and are classified according to their different degrees of concern, ranging from

- ethically unobjectionable (1)
- ethically sensitive (2)
- ethically extremely sensitive (3)
- ethically unacceptable (4)

Each issue is analyzed individually, discussed from different perspectives, and jointly assessed and solved by developing a good attitude of the research group and establishing suitable procedures. In the next step, the identified ethical problems were evaluated and hierarchized according to the four degrees of ethical levels of severity mentioned above. The working session sought to form specific problem clusters from the ethical problem situations identified and hierarchized, which served as a basis for the further solution-oriented procedure. A central goal of the workshop was the creation of a "map" of ethically relevant problem contexts and the joint development of proposed solutions regarding the three dimensions of MEESTAR. Generally, the MEESTAR workshop does not provide answers to ethical questions but instead serves to open a space of reflection within which relevant ethical questions of the "good life" can be thematized, analyzed, and discussed, which have relevance throughout the project period (and partly beyond) regarding the design and functionality of the arrangement. Due to the project's orientation, the contribution of technical assistance systems to an improvement of life (or to the maintenance of the high quality of life) for older target groups was mainly considered and discussed.

7.3 Results

Care
The ethical dimension "care" was relevant for all involved parties—IL associated care mainly with the implications of assistive robotic care on older *people's dignity*. The usage of the system is ethically not justifiable if it compromises the quality of care and if it does not support older people and people in need in maintaining their independence and improving their quality of life while also preserving their potential.

SL associated the impact of a robotic care system on the concept of care, on the one hand, with the *increase of social isolation* and, on the other hand, with the *decrease in commitment and solidarity in families and communities.*

OL expressed ethical concerns regarding marketing and selling interaction as a *commercial product*. From both a social and an organizational perspective, the raised ethical concerns were evaluated as ethically sensitive, which can be compensated for in practice.

Autonomy
The ethical dimension "autonomy" was not a relevant ethical concern for OL. From an individual and social perspective, autonomy was associated primarily with *freedom of choice*. Both perceived the system as a threat to their autonomy if they did not have the *freedom to choose or deny the system,* which was evaluated as ethically extremely sensitive or *forced to use to reduce the care burden on the rest of society.* Latter was only assessed as ethically sensitive.

Safety
IL associated the ethical dimension of safety with implications related to *physical security*. Concerns were made regarding the safe use of the robotic system, especially while food is served directly to the user, e.g., whether the robot can recognize a situation where a patient swallows a meal and needs help. Here, the robot should react appropriately by making an emergency call. This situation would require, therefore, reliable and robust emergency awareness system.

On the one hand, SL associated safety with implications related to *occupational safety*, e.g. *elimination of jobs* that deemed the usage of the system as ethically sensitive. On the other hand, security was also associated with legal protection, including legal liability and safety responsibilities in the case of accidents. If unauthorized data access is detected, rating the system, therefore as ethically extremely sensitive. Hence, relating the ethical principle of safety with the topic of *data security*.

While SL associated safety with occupational safety, OL identified further implications to safety responsibilities of employers and data security, including a *possible competence loss* of the organization through human replacement determining the usage of the system ethically sensitive. OL addressed the concern that workforce skills might shift and change with automation and further *dependency on technology*. This was considered highly morally sensitive.

Privacy
Privacy was associated by all participants, mainly with *data security*, including the possibility of misusing the technology for the *surveillance of users and employers*. SL addressed furthermore the involvement and interest of third parties, such as health-care insurance, in *monitoring the health activities of patients*. This ethical implication was considered ethically sensitive.

Justice
IL related the ethical dimension of justice to *economic concerns*. Concerns were raised over possible *financial criteria that would either exclude people* from using the system or *determine which type of assistance the user should receive*, either technical or personal assistant, rated as incredibly ethically sensitive.

SL discussed the broader social implications in addition to the concerns mentioned above and pointed out that increased use of technical assistance systems could *prevent further political discussions* and hence the social upgrading of these occupational groups. Essentially making it difficult for them to get recognized financially and socially, rating the usage of the system as highly sensitive.

Participation
IL associated the ethical dimension participation with implications related to the quality of interaction addressed already as aspects of the ethical principle autonomy. SL identified furthermore social implications that might result from frequent and sustained human–machine interaction, including the deterioration of social skills such as communications skills which deemed the usage of the system as ethically sensitive. OL pointed out the necessity to include the organization in the decision-making process. There was intense discussion among the participants about the extent to which it is possible and desirable for a technical system to satisfy the need for human interaction and what social implications might result from frequent and sustained human–machine interaction.

Self-conception
Discussion of the ethical dimension of self-conception resulted in similar concerns listed already as implications of the aforementioned dimensions.

7.4 Discussion

The quality of life should not only be considered from an individual perspective. Still, it should instead be socially negotiated and communicated to understand what can be mutually expected and what is seen as the standard of social cohesion.

All participants agreed that it is neither desirable nor intended to replace interpersonal relationships completely and human care with human–machine relationships since the quality of human care and relationships cannot be technically simulated. It should not be substituted provided further desirable development of society. The consortium assessed the integration of social and communicative skills critically for several reasons and rejected it for two reasons. First, integrating social and communicative functions into the system creates a social bond or a user's dependency on the system. Second, the system should be prevented from influencing the user's opinion-forming and decision-making processes through standardized communication modules or adaptive functions that adjust to the user's interests—especially concerning the vulnerability of the target group and the possible cognitive impairments, the risk that an intensive social relationship developing between the user and the system could contribute to users forgetting that they are interacting with a technical design. Language capabilities should only be present so that purpose-bound communication is possible.

In this context, a distinction between "helping and assisting" that Prof. Manzeschke has elaborated might prove helpful.

Help is a *person-to-person activity* in which one person makes their resources, abilities, or self-available to another to achieve the goals, which the latter can no longer do on their own. *Assistance* is the *technical simulation and substitution of help*. It contains the functional element of human help without the "admixture" of the social aspect of the human encounter. This is partly experienced as very relieving. Technical assistance ranges from simple aids to complex technical arrangements. With the help of this fundamental distinction, it is possible to precisely target what the system should and should not do and which form—help or assistance—is necessary, desirable, or preferable in which situation is essential, desirable, or preferable in which situation is necessary, desirable, or preferable in which case. Regardless of this general attitude, however, the question was raised to what extent the act of eating is a social practice whose social elements would be eliminated by reducing it to a purely functional interaction of preparing and enriching food. This could, under certain circumstances, be perceived as a deterioration of the quality of life of the persons concerned—especially if the fact is considered that the use of the robot leads to a reduction of the presence of the caregiver.

The project team agreed that the robot's functions must always be transparent. Complete and accessible information for consumers will be necessary when the system is introduced to the market. Strategies include creating detailed, easy-to-understand instructions explaining the product's usage and specification for the different user groups. In addition, there was a widespread agreement that the technical system should not be sold to vulnerable groups as a stand-alone, "unattended" system, as constant and competent monitoring and assessment were necessary concerning the user's competence. Nevertheless, the question arose as to whether and how knowledge of the user's loss of ability could be obtained, as the user may not be willing to disclose due to shame or fear of failure, the user may not be ready to reveal that they are having problems using the system. At the same time, they are frustrated that they can no longer use the system autonomously. This resulted in the discussion of the ethically relevant question of how to deal with persons who once had the technical design but then, due to cognitive or performative loss of ability from the assisted care.

The following distinction between models of use and distribution might serve as a basis for answering those questions:

1. The assistance system is distributed as a stand-alone device. This would allow any potentially interested party to purchase, install, and use the device unaccompanied (Dyadic model).
2. The device is installed under the supervision of a competent technician and is tailored to the needs and abilities of the individual user. This also mainly includes questions of the range of functions, in the case of a modularized solution, and questions of the inclusion of third parties in the interaction between user and system (Extended dyadic model with the potential inclusion of third parties).
3. The use of the device is made possible exclusively in combination with a supervising person who is informed about the user's competencies in dealing with the system and over their possibly undesired emotional occupation of the system (Triadic Model).

7.5 Conclusion

The *RoPHa* project aims at supporting care-dependent people to lead a more independent life in the context of food intake. To advance the design and acceptability of socially interactive robots, it is necessary to evaluate the ethical implications of our envisioned technical assistance systems. The MEESTAR model was explicitly designed to provide an ethical evaluation of socio-technical arrangements. It determines the impact of such agreement concerning their design and functionality based on concrete scenarios. The evaluation aided in the identification of ethically relevant problems as well as in the joint development of proposed solutions. This could lead to undesirable social consequences regarding expectations and trust in the system. On the one hand, users could overestimate the robot's capabilities and inevitably experience frustrations if the robot cannot provide the desired functionality, empathy, and support. On the other hand, a social trust relationship opens the possibility of the technical system influencing the user's decision-making processes.

The discussion focused mainly on whether the consortium should actively contribute to creating an emotional and social bond between the user and the technical system, e.g., through design decisions and decisions regarding the system's functionality emerge between the user and the technological system. The consortium believes that the decision to use the system should be made only with the user's consent to ensure that the user perceives the system as helpful support and not as an unwanted or frightening coercive measure. It was a consensus that technical safety would have to be ensured to avoid accidents. Regardless of this objective, there would always be a residual risk of technical failure or technical dysfunctionality. The user should be informed in advance in an understandable, comprehensible form of possible threats to compensate for this.

The topic of security was discussed in its various facets. Particular attention was paid to the idea of monitoring all participants collaborating with the robot. To avoid profound ethical implications, it was agreed that it is necessary to define early in the system design how data will be collected, processed, and stored in RoPHa. Furthermore, the user should be informed in an understandable and accessible form about the collection and storage of data and should own the option of terminating the use of the system at any time. The principle of data economy and local data storage should apply to the research context to minimize the ever-present risk of data misuse.

The evaluation based on the MEESTAR model proved significantly as it made it possible to define a clear role for a care robot, including defining social, communicative, and technical capabilities.

References

Eurosat. (2020). *Aging in Europe – Looking at the lives of older people in the EU - 2020 edition*. Publications Office of the European Union. https://doi.org/10.2785/628105

Manzeschke A, Weber K, Rother E, & Fangerau H (2015). *Ethical questions in the area of age appropriate assisting systems*. Druckerei Thiel Gruppe. Retrieved January 27, 2022 from https://www.researchgate.net/publication/304743219_Ethical_questions_in_the_area_of_age_appropriate_assisting_systems

Mona Abdel-Keream, M.Sc., is a Ph.D. student under the supervision of Prof. Michael Beetz. She has a master's degree in Biomedical Engineering (2017) from the University of Applied Sciences of Vienna. She pursued her master thesis project in the Artificial Hands Lab at the Biorobotics Institute of the Sant' Anna University (Italy). Since December 2017, she has been a member of the Artificial Institute of the University of Bremen. She works on simulation-based methods, using Game Engines and Virtual Reality for robotic assistive applications, and is particularly interested in studying and designing knowledge-based models for intelligent and aware household robots.

Open Access This chapter is licensed under the terms of the Creative Commons Attribution 4.0 International License (http://creativecommons.org/licenses/by/4.0/), which permits use, sharing, adaptation, distribution and reproduction in any medium or format, as long as you give appropriate credit to the original author(s) and the source, provide a link to the Creative Commons license and indicate if changes were made.

The images or other third party material in this chapter are included in the chapter's Creative Commons license, unless indicated otherwise in a credit line to the material. If material is not included in the chapter's Creative Commons license and your intended use is not permitted by statutory regulation or exceeds the permitted use, you will need to obtain permission directly from the copyright holder.

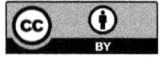

GPSR Compliance
The European Union's (EU) General Product Safety Regulation (GPSR) is a set of rules that requires consumer products to be safe and our obligations to ensure this.

If you have any concerns about our products, you can contact us on

ProductSafety@springernature.com

In case Publisher is established outside the EU, the EU authorized representative is:

Springer Nature Customer Service Center GmbH
Europaplatz 3
69115 Heidelberg, Germany

www.ingramcontent.com/pod-product-compliance
Ingram Content Group UK Ltd.
Pitfield, Milton Keynes, MK11 3LW, UK
UKHW021957040925
462611UK00004B/448